Barbara Simonsohn

Barley Grass Juice

Rejuvenation Elixir
and Natural, Healthy Power Drink

Easy to Prepare and Totally Healthy, Barley Grass Juice
Works True Wonders
A Perfect Food with a
Complete Complex of Vital Substances

Translated by Christine M. Grimm

T0095010

LOTUS PRESS
SHANGRI-LA

Important Note

The information presented in this book has been carefully researched and passed on to our best knowledge and conscience. Despite this fact, neither the author nor the publisher assume any type of liability for presumed or actual damages of any kind that might result from the direct or indirect application or use of the statements in this book.

The information in this book is solely intended for interested readers and educational purposes and should in no way be understood as diagnostic or therapeutic instructions in the medical sense. If you suspect the existence of an illness, we definitely recommend that you see a physician or healing practitioner and expressly discourage you from diagnosing and treating yourself.

First English Edition 2001
© by Lotus Press, Box 325
Twin Lakes, WI 53181, USA
The Shangri-La Series is published in cooperation with Schneeloewe Verlagsberatung, Federal Republic of Germany
© 1999 by Windpferd Verlagsgesellschaft mbH, Aitrang, Germany
All rights reserved
Translated by Christine M. Grimm
Illustrations
Pg. 4: Ulla Mayer-Raichle
Pg. 9, 16, 23, 27, 32, 55–57, 59, 89: Theo Hodapp
Pg. 8, 12, 14, 48, 63–66: Green Foods Corporation, Europe
Pg. 39: Doris Diekelmann from *Heilpflanzen der Bibel*, Windpferd Verlag, Aitrang, Germany
Pg. 44, 45: Ann Wigmore Institute
Pg. 55: by Green Foods, Oxnard, CA, USA
Pg. 125, 127, 128: Schneeloewe Picture
Cover design by Kuhn Grafik, Digitales Design, Zurich
Using a photo by Ulla Mayer-Raichle
Overall production: Schneeloewe, Aitrang, Germany

ISBN 0-914955-68-3
Library of Congress Control Number 2001132217

Printed in USA

Table of Contents

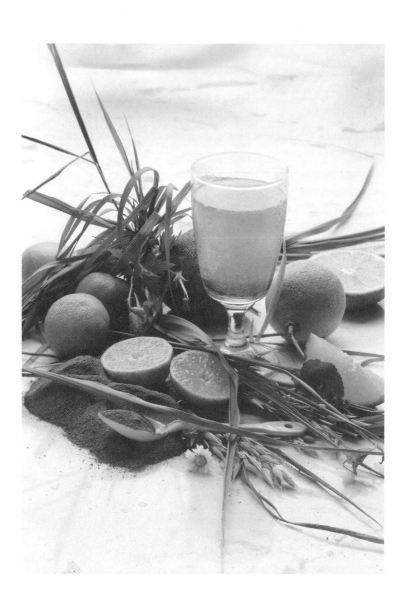

ACKNOWLEDGEMENTS

Many people have once again contributed their love, time, and energy to the creation of this book. My thanks and recognition go to my German publisher, Monika Jünemann, who has supported me in writing about a book topic that was still "untouched" in the German-language area, as well as to author Halima Neumann, who spent many hours reading my manuscript. She gave me numerous valuable tips and suggestions, in addition to some barley grass recipes. I would also like to thank my friend Brit for her research and development of tasty and healthy recipes with barley grass. In addition, I would like to thank author Harald Tietze of Australia for making the documentation for his book *Green Medicine*, with its many reports on experiences by barley grass users, available to me. I would also like to thank my children Freya and Michael for testing the recipes and barley grass tablets and giving me their friendly but assertive opinions as to whether they were delicious or not.

I thank Dr. Mary Ruth Swope, Dr. Yoshihide Hagiwara, and Dr. Ann Wigmore, health pioneers who inspired me through their books on the health advantages of barley grass and other cereal grasses. They enthused me about the topic for this book. Their books express a deep love of humanity and the belief that we can free ourselves from our current health problems if we reconnect with the power of nature and the will of the Creator.

A special thanks to Bob Terry from Green Foods Corporation in Oxnard, CA for reviewing the manuscript and for giving helpful suggestions and comments. Furthermore, I would like to thank Ms. Lebrato of the German *Allcura* company for proofreading some of the chapters and Mr. Van de Kelder of the *Green Foods Corporation Europe* in Brussels for making the scientific studies on the health advantages of Green Magma, a barley grass powder, and extensive photographic material available to me. In addition, I thank *Pines International* and *Wakunaga of America* in the USA; *Arise & Shine*, *Fitness 2000*, and the *Melrose Company* of Australia; and *Bionika Versand, Keimling Naturkost, Papaya Vera, Pura Vita, Positive Produkte, Sanos GbR, Sanatur, Spira Verde Versand* in Europe for the background information about barley grass and their barley grass products. At this point, I would also like to thank the German organic farmer and philosopher Baldur Springmann for his contribution on the wonder of photosynthesis. I thank the *Living Food Institute* in Sweden for the valuable information on wheat grass treatments, as well as the English-language books by Dr. Ann Wigmore. In addition, I thank Theo Hodapp for his loving support and patience during the computer problems, as well as the "overtime" he put in caring for our two children during the final phase of this book.

INTRODUCTION

More than twenty years ago, I was at the Findhorn Community in the northern part of Scotland for the first time. Findhorn is a spiritual community in which holistic approaches to healing are taught and lived.

Sunday morning, as everyone else seemed to be asleep, I went into the kitchen of Cluny Hill College to make myself some herbal tea. As I opened the swinging door, I was quite surprised to meet someone this early—it was shortly after 6 o'clock: David, an attractive Israeli who I had met the day before in a workshop. I greeted him and was surprised to see him apparently stuffing grass into a silver-colored meat grinder. Batches of dark-green juice were flowing out of it and into a bowl. "What are you doing?," I asked him in surprise. "Oh," he said somewhat embarrassed, "I'm just making myself some barley grass juice." "And why?" Then David told me that he had stomach cancer. But since he started drinking freshly squeezed barley grass juice every day, he was completely free of any symptoms. "As soon as I become forgetful and lazy and stop drinking the barley grass juice, the cancer becomes noticeable again!" he said with a sunny smile.

I learned that David, before he came to Findhorn, had asked a friend in London to grow barley grass on the windowsill for him. Then, on the way to Findhorn, David had harvested these "fields of barley grass" while stopping at his friend's place. He packed it in plastic bags and took it along to Findhorn. He had been provided with a refrigerator for storing the barley grass there. This made it possible for him to extract a small glass of barley grass juice in a hand-operated wheat grass juicer, which I had mistakenly thought was a meat grinder, every day.

Cereal Grasses—A Cure for Cancer and Therapy against Addiction

David told me a great deal about the health advantages of grass juices. And he gave me the telephone number of Dr. Ann Wigmore, who had become famous because of her barley grass and wheat grass juice treatments for cancer patients and drug-addicted youth at her Hippocrates Health Institute in Boston. Since this time, I have grown barley grass and wheat grass on my windowsill. I enjoy the rich, green juice, which is not only a refreshing sight to the eye but also beneficial for the body and soul.

In the USA, there are many vegetarian restaurants, wellness hotels, health food stores, natural food stores, and juice bars where people can drink truly *fresh*-squeezed fruit and vegetable juices, as well as fresh barley grass juice and wheat grass juice.

This may not be the case in other countries, but anyone can have fun growing these grasses at home or while on vacation. It's quite simple. In addition, dried barley grass is also available for purchase as a powder to mix or in tablet form in health food stores and natural food stores, as well as through mail-order companies. To make this high quality, natural food supplement, organically grown grain is harvested at the time of the greatest nutrient concentration. This occurs shortly before the stam formation, which is also called the jointing stage. Although processing techniques vary, the ideal way is to wash and extract the juice as fast as possible, using no chemicals or heat, and then to gently spray-dry the juice so that the juice nutrients are not heated above body temperature.

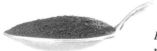

In Japan, barley grass powder is already the most popular food supplement

Barley Grass Extract:
Nature's Best "Fast Food"

Dr. Yoshihide Hagiwara, the discoverer of barley grass calls barley grass powder "nature's best fast food." The barley grass powder that he has patented, Green Magma, is the best-selling food supplement in Japan and is already a best-seller in the USA as well.

Simply mix the green powder, which smells and tastes like spinach or grass, with non-carbonated water. If the taste is too boring for you, you can also mix it with banana, grape, pineapple, or pear juice (if possible, from organic cultivation) and mix a teaspoon of blue-green algae powder into the juice. Anyone, even those who don't have the desire or time to grow the grass at home, can therefore still profit from the many health advantages of barley grass!

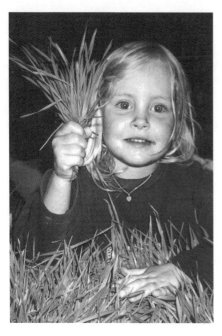

A supply of vital substances like barley grass juice (or extract) protects our children against disease and provides their bodies with everything that they need to strengthen its defensive and self-healing powers

Barley grass juice is not only a potent healing remedy, as David plausibly demonstrated to me at Findhorn; it also prevents nutritionally-caused diseases by providing the body with vital substances that are no longer adequately present in our foods. The body's powers sof self-healing are strengthened, the ability to deal with stress increases, and the body is supported in helping protect itself against the germs of disease.

A HOLISTIC FOOD TO SOLVE OUR NUTRITIONAL PROBLEMS

Our Nutrient Deficits Are Becoming Serious

The costs of nutritionally caused diseases in Germany are estimated to be very high. In the United States the situation is even more dramatic. The American population has the highest pro capita spending for health care in the world but they are only number 27 on the list of industrial nations with the longest life expectancy. This is not only horrifying in terms of the economy, but also reveals the health misery of the millions who suffer from chronic diseases like arteriosclerosis, cancer, rheumatism, multiple sclerosis, or diabetes. Dying of old age has almost become a rarity: Most people die from some form of disease.

People are "starving in front of full pots" today in view of the widespread poor nutrition and inadequate supplies of vital substances. Furthermore, there is an insidious, hardly noticeable nutritional plight: apples only contain 20% of the vitamin C, fennel only one-fifth as much beta carotene, broccoli only one-third as much calcium, and carrots barely half as much magnesium as they did just ten years ago. The situation is no better for other types of fruits and vegetables.[1] The blame for this can be found in the worn-out soil, the long transportation distances and storage, and the way that food is overcooked on our own stoves. At the same time, because of our increasingly disturbing living conditions like stress, smog, and noise pollution, we now need *more* vital substances than ten years ago.

Knowledge about the significance of nutrients and nutritional supplements with preventive and therapeutic qualities is slowly increasing in the general public—and not just among scientists and authors of books who deal with these topics. The will to have a healthy lifestyle is already surprisingly widespread; however, most people are lacking in the motivation to also practice this increased level of knowledge in everyday life. Convenience and the nutritional habits that we have been brought up with—and which are cemented in place by the advertising world, seem to create an insurmountable obstacle on the path to a healthier life for many people. Barley grass extract, which is easily available and can be prepared in a matter of seconds, could change this situation and lead to a positive spiral: The more vital substances we absorb, the more power we have to decide on a healthy lifestyle.

In the press, "antioxidants" play a large role in the prevention of disease and delay of the aging processes. The U.S. Department of Agriculture writes in its recommendations of 1995 that the antioxidant nutrients in foods of a plant origin (like vitamin C, vitamin E, carotene, and the mineral selenium), have become of great interest to scientists and also for the public because of their use to reduce the risk of becoming ill with cancer and other chronic diseases.

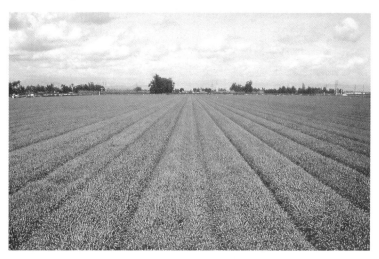

The more vital substances we absorb, the more power we have—pure vital substances in the most perfect form are only supplied by Mother Nature

Synthetically Produced Vitamins and Mineral Substances Become Problematic

Many nutritional supplements contain only a few isolated nutrients, often synthetic, whereas whole plants contain hundreds of different substances including essential nutrients and potentially beneficial phytochemicals. But plants have hundreds of active substances that have not yet been discovered. These combine in a very complex manner and work as mutual catalysts, creating reciprocally supportive synergistic effects. If we take just one or two isolated vitamins or minerals, this may cause an imbalance in our entire vitamin and mineral household.

Synthetically produced vitamins and minerals have increasingly become a controversial issue. For chemists, ascorbic acid and the vitamin C of acerola cherries are chemically the same substance. However, artificial and isolated vitamin C is metabolized in a completely different manner by the body and can lead to such disorders as allergies.

In addition to well known carotenoids, beta-carotene, lutein, and lycopene, more than 600 different carotenoids have now been identified in plants. Yet, the commercially available beta carotene preparations contain a maximum of three. Studies in the USA and Norway in which former smokers were given beta carotene preparations had to be discontinued because the participants developed a greater risk of lung cancer than the average former smoker. Eating just one carrot a day can reduce your risk of cancer by forty percent! Isolated preparations are lacking in nutrients like vitamins, bioflavonoids, enzymes, and trace elements, which create a reciprocally supportive synergistic effect and/or make the functioning of the vital substance possible in the first place. The body utilizes foods that exist in nature much more completely: we could call this the optimal "biological availability."

Barley Grass Extract has a High Level of Biological Availability

Barley grass extract in powder or tablet form is a *holistic food concentrate of natural origin*. It contains all the nutrients and phyto-chemicals of the green barley grass in their natural proportions. The wholeness of barley grass is what makes it such an effective food and healing remedy. The individual components such as enzymes, minerals, and vitamins work together in this living, enzyme-active food in a synergistic manner ("the whole is more than the sum of its parts"). The result is the intensification of their positive effects on our health.

Barley grass extract contains all of the nutrients that are found in organically grown barley grass in their natural proportions and in the state in which Mother Nature created them.

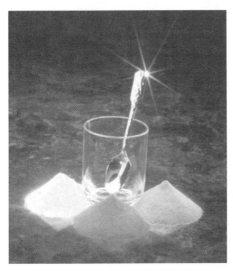

Barley grass extract is a whole food of natural origin—both an effective food and healing remedy

An abundance of scientific studies on the health advantages of barley grass extract have been collected through the decades, thanks above all to the untiring activities of Dr. Yoshihide Hagiwara. Ten percent of the proceeds from "Green Magma", which he developed and patented, are invested in further research projects.

Deficiencies in vital substances are pre-programmed in the types of foods that most people eat. Taking multivitamins or multi-mineral tablets from the drug store or pharmacy is a questionable solution to this problem. According to my experience, it is not possible to improve upon nature. Has a human being ever created a living cell, a plant, or an animal in a laboratory? No. If we want to prevent disease or premature aging processes and experience true vitality and joy in life, it is necessary to additionally provide the body with concentrated food supplements of a natural origin, such as barley grass powder.

Chlorophyll, the Blood of Plants

What Makes the Grass so Green?

One of the first people to discover an answer to this question was the European chemist Richard Willstaetter (1872-1942) who received the Nobel Prize in Chemistry for his research results in 1935. He found out that chlorophyll, the green pigment of plants, consists of two components: the blue-green chlorophyll of type A and the yellow-green chlorophyll of type B in a proportion of about three to one.

Both types of chlorophyll are related to the red blood pigment hemin, with the sole difference that chlorophyll contains magnesium and the hemin molecule contains iron at its molecular center. Dr. Yoshihide Hagiwara says that chlorophyll and blood appear to be twins in their chemical structure. Hemin connects with globin, a protein, and thereby forms hemoglobin, which is found in the red blood corpuscles and is also called "blood pigment."

Chlorophyll is considered to be the blood-forming element of nature for all herbivores and human beings. Within a plant, chlorophyll is used as stored sun energy for new organic syntheses for life processes. Halima Neumann* states that chlorophyll is the only substance that can pass on the stored sun energy through the food to the human cell. The knowledgeable barley grass enthusiasts, Dr. Mary Ruth Swope and Dr. Yoshihide Hagiwara believe that the "green blood" of the plants can be transformed into red blood in the human body: The fluid in the green leaves represents the blood of the grasses and trees. Consequently, chlorophyll also works as quickly as iron in animals and human beings with anemia. It is important to remember that the formation of blood depends not only on chlorophyll: the vitamins C, B12, K, A, folic acid, and pyridoxine, also contained in barley grass, are important for the creation of healthy blood as well.

---

* Halima Neumann is a well-known nutrition pioneer and author of various health books in German language.

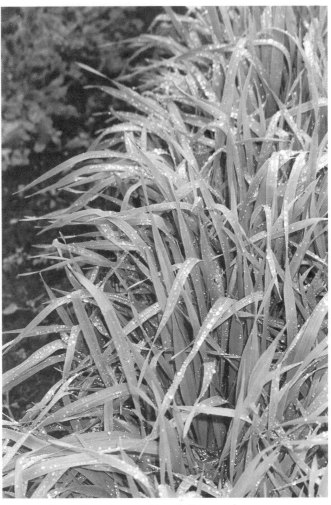

Green plant pigment, chlorophyll, is stored sun energy

Chlorophyll is the Basis of All Life

Without this green plant pigment, life could not exist on earth because there would be no food to eat and no oxygen to breathe. With photosynthesis, chlorophyll is responsible for transforming the carbon dioxide that animals and human beings exhale, as well as being constantly produced by industry and traffic, back into oxygen. This is why it is so important to preserve our "green lungs," the rainforests in South America. However, these are being burned down and cleared at an increasing tempo for subsistence farmers and—to a much greater extent—to create the pampas upon which the cattle for hamburger chains in the USA and Europe can graze. Living without meat or limiting its consumption would be an important step in assuming responsibility for this dramatic situation. Incidentally, numerous scientific studies have now proved that vegetarians lead healthier lives.

Dr. Yoshihide Hagiwara criticizes the fact that Japan "imports" about two-thirds of its required oxygen from the Amazon delta. This naturally occurs without payment or an exchange of energy because much more oxygen is used in Japan than is produced as a result of overpopulation and industrialization. The situation is similar in other places.

But there are organizations such as the Rainforest Action Network, The Rainforest Alliance, and the World Rainforest Movement that are committed to preserving the rainforest, upon whose oxygen production we depend. These organizations can be supported by working for them and/or making financial donations to them. There are more than 600,000 pages related to the tropical rainforest on the Internet! Many organizations arrange environmentally-friendly trips, label environmentally-tolerable products, provide lists of such products, and support research projects for the preservation of the rainforest and its inhabitants. They also develop educational units for teachers and projects for students of all age groups. These organizations support local environmental groups in the tropical belt of our planet, as well as ecological agriculture and horticulture. By becoming involved with these organizations, we can do something for our future and our children's future.

Chlorophyll Forms Blood and Strengthens Every Organ

When chlorophyll from plants is absorbed by the body, it not only serves as an important source of magnesium but it may also increase the formation of the oxygen-carrier, hemoglobin. Green juices and green vegetables like wild herbs are therefore an excellent possibility for preventing and healing anemia (iron deficiency), from which about 60% of the women in industrial nations suffer. Magnesium strengthens our nervous system and muscle tissue, which means it is the most important mineral for maintaining a healthy heart and respiratory activity up into old age. A lack of magnesium in our worn-out and over-fertilized soil represents a worldwide health risk for the animals and human beings who must pay for it with muscle atrophy and heart diseases.

Chlorophyll-containing foods may also increase the formation of the oxygen-carrier, hemoglobin, thereby providing the body's cells with a greater supply of oxygen. Through this increased supply of oxygen, cell division is accelerated, metabolic processes are optimized, and the brain cells receive better blood circulation, making them more efficient. Chlorophyll helps the body in its necessary repair work; examples of this are injuries or burns. Barley grass and blue-green algae juice instead of acid-forming coffee as the first meal of the day are recommended by nutrition experts.

Without exception, every organ is strengthened and harmonized by the green-colored pigment. Among other organs, the heart, the immune system, and the eyes are strengthened by chlorophyll. Green also plays a large role in color therapy: The color green calms, harmonizes, heals the body and soul, and therefore stands for the principle of hope, renewal, and rejuvenation. The green plant pigment, which is created through photosynthesis, has a concentration of sunlight and the power of the sun and its light.

In the spiritual sense, the sun is the symbol of wisdom (light) and unconditional love (warmth). The color green is associated with the heart chakra, one of our main energy centers. Through green food and walks in the green of nature, we can develop our heart chakra. We are invited to connect with the powers of love and wisdom through the green plant food and profit from them [also see "Barley Grass from the Spiritual Perspective" (pages 33 ff.) and the essay by the German organic farmer and philosopher Baldur Springmann on the topic of photosynthesis (page 23 ff.)]

Synergetic Effects of Barley Grass

The topic of the "synergetic effects of nutrients" has already been touched upon in the chapter on "The Significance of Grass Juices for Our Health" on pages 27 ff. This also applies to chlorophyll from natural sources. The trace elements of iron and copper from green plants effectively enrich the blood because iron can only be deposited in the hemoglobin together with a supply of copper. Even when there is an adequate supply of iron, a copper deficiency often leads to gray hair and anemia! Copper from "green food" is essential for color-pigment formation in the skin and hair. It has been determined that the simultaneous administration of chlorophyll and iron increases the number of red corpuscles and raises the level of hemoglobin more quickly than taking iron by itself. Chemically produced chlorophyll does not have the same effect, the biochemical activity of natural chlorophyll is lost, and even negative side effects like anemia or nausea may occur.[2]

Since many supplements contain only isolated nutrients, mostly of synthetic origin, they lack the abundant support nutrients and factors normally present in whole foods. Because of this, the body does not utilize these supplements efficiently, or even safely. The same also applies to other isolated plant vitamin or mineral preparations. The fatal consequences of this: When taken over a longer period of time and at high dosages, synthetically produced or isolated substances not in their original complete form often have a negative and toxic effect. This can manifest itself through nausea, constipation, fatigue, or headaches.

Isolated substances are stored in the connective tissue and inner organs like the liver. Such dangers do not exist for green plant foods like algae, fresh plant juices, green grass juices, or extracts like barley grass powder or the Egyptian primal wheat grass kamut because the body easily eliminates any excess.

Barley Grass Supplies Calcium

Chlorophyll-containing plant foods have a great deal of calcium, which can only be used by the body in an organically balanced compound with magnesium. Calcium is important for the strengthening of bones, cartilage, and supporting tissue—and can prevent osteoporosis. In our modern age, even children suffer from deossification (softening of the bones). The main cause is seen in the increasing consumption of soft drinks, which contain the calcium-depleting agent phosphoric acid. Despite all the praise it receives, milk is unsuitable as a supplier of calcium since it does not contain magnesium and calcium absorption cannot be guaranteed without magnesium. In areas such as the USA and Europe, where the consumption of milk products is constantly increasing, osteoporosis is a major problem, above all, for older women. However, in countries where there is very little consumption of milk products, this ailment is a rarity.

Moreover, chlorophyll-containing green juices like barley grass juice regenerate the intestinal flora, the digestive organs, and the entire endocrine hormone-producing gland system because of their abundance of enzymes. Digestion and food utilization are optimized as a result. In addition, chlorophyll has a germ-killing effect.

Chlorophyll Strengthens the Powers of Resistance

With green juices like barley grass juice or powder, we stimulate our powers of resistance so that we are increasingly better protected against infectious diseases. This is especially important in an age where the strains of bacteria are becoming resistant to antibiotics.

In addition, chlorophyll improves the brain functions and can lower the cholesterol level, which is one of the causes of heart attack and stroke. The proteins and other substances in chlorophyll-containing plants an anti-inflammatory effect and can even interrupt the cycle of a disease once it has begun by creating the preconditions for healing. Dr. Yoshihide Hagiwara reports about his severe skin inflammation, caused by boiling water, which he was able to heal by just applying the juice from green barley.

The enzymes such as superoxide dismutase (SOD) and catalase found in barley grass can prevent and also heal cancer. There is more information about this in the chapter "Barley Grass Against Cancer" on page 108. Enzymes may also be the substances responsible for barley grass' ability to effectively degrade toxins like organophosphate-containing pesticides.

Chlorophyll Strengthens the Powers of Self-Healing

The effect of chlorophyll is not limited to specific health disorders but strengthens the overall powers of self-healing and natural regulation mechanisms of the organism. Dr. Yoshihide Hagiwara postulates that a substance (meaning barley grass extract, author's note) that is effective against obesity and eczema, as well as heart diseases and cancer, is either an incredible "wonder remedy" or absolutely not a medication but something that promotes true healing wonders—meaning the ability of the body to heal itself.

Moreover, the enzyme complexes have antioxidant effects: They even fight the free radicals, aggressive oxygen molecules, and consequently prevent cell degeneration and aging, as well as the development of chronic diseases like cancer.

It has even been suggested that green grass juices provide protection against radioactive damage caused by radiation from sources such as x-rays. However, all of these beneficial effects of the chlorophyll on the harmonization and normalization of the body functions only occur when it is taken on a regular, daily basis. Furthermore, the effect of the enzymes, vitamins, and minerals must not be destroyed or decimated by heating them. This is why only fresh green vegetables, kitchen or wild herbs, freshly pressed green juices from barley grass, for example, or extracts like barley grass or blue-green algae powder in a raw-food quality should be considered for this purpose when we want to get as much benefit as possible from the advantages of chlorophyll for our health.

The true "green revolution," the appreciation and intake of more green, chlorophyll containing plants, is still ahead!

Photosynthesis
and Protein Formation in the Plant

"Are you seeking the Highest, the Greatest? The plant can teach you! What it will-lessly is, you should want to become! This is it." (FRIEDRICH SCHILLER)

Many years ago, I "coincidentally" met Baldur Springmann on a train trip from Cologne to Hamburg. I was so fascinated by his message, his clarity and charisma, that I spontaneously decided to live and learn at the "Hof Springe"—the organic-dynamic farm near Bad Segeberg, Germany, for a year. In the following section of this book, Baldur has provided an article that first appeared in edition number 72/94 of the *Raum & Zeit* German-language magazine (and is printed in a shortened version here). I thank Baldur Springmann for this inspiring contribution!

Guest Article by Baldur Springmann

(Organic Farmer and Philosopher)

A Marriage Between Heaven and Earth Occurs Constantly in the Chlorophyll Grains

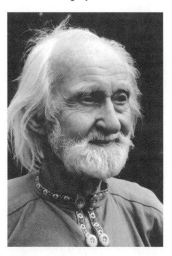

Baldur Springmann is among the pioneers of the German natural foods movement. He is a man who lives what he teaches, and this includes the spiritual dimension of food in particular.

Although it may appear to be without a will when compared to other beings, our sister the plant shows us that the polarity, this law of the world in earthly life, is manifested in a special form. On the scale of ecology, giving and taking are not equal and invariable constants. When we take a closer look, there is a tendency to recognize one development, which gives increasingly more predominance to one side since giving increasing develops into something more.

Yes, it's true! Just take a more precise look at something like the generally known **process of photosynthesis**! The chemical formula, which is actually required knowledge for every person who wants to protect the life on this planet, says that in each of the countless many green leaves is an entire multitude of green-glassy churches in which constantly, day in and day out, and therefore directly in front of our frequently blind eyes, a wonder occurs. These are the chlorophyll grains in which the marriage of heaven and earth is constantly celebrated—and in the following manner.

The earthly substances of oxygen (O), which we could more accurately call "the substance of life," and carbon (C), which we could more accurately call "the substance of the earth," are inhaled by the leaf in the form of carbon dioxide. If human beings have not polluted this air, this substance is found in a very specific ratio within this mixture of gases. In addition, these substances reach the leaf through the roots in the form of water. And here is where they embrace a child of light that the sun has sent them. The result of this embrace is glucose, which can later develop into starch—precisely the same starch that we eat in our daily bread. So it should be clear to us that we also eat a heavenly gift from the dear sun, in addition to the substances of the earth, air, and life, with each bite of bread!

This "child of light" that is immanent to the starch should be described in greater detail here. An extensive treatise would be required on the spiritual reality of "light," of which Goethe already (or still!) knew that—like all things spiritual, it cannot be seen by our eyes nor measured by our instruments. All the things that we can see and measure are just the "deeds and suffering of the light," as he called it.

The Magic Wand of Chlorophyll Allows the Sun's Energy to Become Life Energy

One of the "deeds," one of the many qualities in which the spiritual fact of light manifests itself for us is energy. So we can also measure it and know as a result that 645 kcal are gathered into one single molecule of starch. We also know that this is the only and the unique form of energy that keeps the entire pendulum of life in earth in motion, every beat of a bird's wing, every bat of an eyelash, every breath, and every beat of our heart, everything that exists.

Doesn't it make us totally humble to think everything was originally a gift of the sun? Or have any of us ever received a bill for such and such many calories? In addition, the entire system is not set up in the same short-circuited way that human engineers would have used to create it: sun energy simply, snap, into the animal, through the skin or something like that, and then fill up the muscle machine with this power drink. No, the cosmic intelligence has provided the **monopoly of the green leaves** for this purpose. **The magic wand of chlorophyll** is only present in the chlorophyll grains alone, allowing the sun's energy to become life energy—and in a much larger amount than would be necessary for the respective plant by itself. This makes it possible for the plant to pass it on to everything that creeps on the earth and flies and swims and buzzes.

The photosynthesis of the plant, which allows oxygen to be created from carbon dioxide, is a chemical formula plus a miracle: $6\ CO_2 + 12\ H_2O + 645\ kcal + 1$ miracle $= C_6H_{12}O_6 + 6\ H_2O + 6\ O_2$. On top of all this, this giving is so much fun for the plant that it produces much more than the animals need. Through millions of years, Mother Earth has carefully stored this excess in her coal and oil storage chamber, definitely not for the purpose of humanity now cashing in on all of it within a short time.

The Plant Makes Valuable Protein from Nitrogen

There is so much in this story that could make us become even more pious. I could keep telling it until tomorrow morning. If some of you shake your heads at me because I go into raptures about it, then I will cheerfully also admit that tears have often welled up in my eyes when I leaned against a birch tree and dreamily looked up into its leaves. And I hardly dare to relate the second story, the one about the **protein** that is just as indispensable for our nourishment as the starch. You will soon notice why. You are certain to know that this protein is also synthesized within the plants. And, in turn, there is an astonishing fact here as well: namely, although nitrogen (N) is the element that determines the nature of the hundreds of thousands of atoms in the artfully designed protein molecule and constitutes 78% of the air we breathe, neither our lungs nor the plants can absorb and utilize it.

Once again, the one-track human mind sees this circumstance to be "hair-raising" since the most "rational" approach has not been taken: introducing the excess atmospheric nitrogen, snap, directly into the developing protein. But, no way. This situation is even more unusual than that of photosynthesis. In this case, only certain strains of bacteria that live in the humus absorb the nitrogen from the air and can build them into the amino acids and protein substances. From what is left behind, the saltpeter and ammonia salts are formed in the soil. The plant roots can then drink these solutions, including the nitrogen that is contained in them.

In my opinion, the contemporary ethos should be considerably more supported by the type of togetherness that the Creation reveals to us when we look at it with open hearts and the astonished researcher eyes of the ecologist.

In response to these statements, the editors of the magazine *Raum & Zeit* have commented that this essay—which imparts so much heart and understanding for our surrounding world and ourselves—should actually be read in every school at on the first day, at every university when the semester begins, and in every church at the beginning of the church year. This essay contains the most important part of the legacy of a very wise man.

Grass Juices for Our Health

Rye, wheat, barley, corn, oats, and sugarcane all belong to the family of grasses. It is astonishing that human beings have used grain and grass seeds as food for thousands of years but have overlooked the nourishment that the grasses themselves offer. Cereal grass is a complete food. Because of its protective and healing value, it should be included in our diets[3].

Author Ronald Seibold's opinion, the significance of all dark-green vegetables in our diets cannot be emphasized enough. Since cereal grasses are concentrated green foods, he thinks it is important to include them in addition to the dark-green leafy types of vegetables in our daily diets.[4]

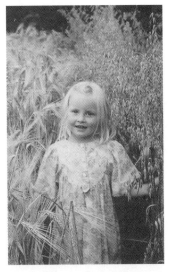

Grain offers an almost non-perishable, storable food, but its grass juices are an incomparable fresh source of vital substances

Dr. Ann Wigmore tells of a prophecy made thousands of years ago on the sunken continent of Atlantis. This prophecy said that a far distant civilization will one day receive a "key" in the form of cereal grass that will preserve a decayed civilization from becoming extinct. Does this perhaps refer to our generation?

Grass Juices Protect Us Against Crises

The value of the grass-juice factor in the food of human beings is not yet generally known. But what science has already discovered about the health value of grass juices should convince us that we must include these juices in our diets in order to promote our mental and physical health.

Viktoras Kulvinskas, formerly a computer scientist and mathematician at Harvard University and now a well-known health evangelist says that those who drink grass juice in these critical times are better armed to survive ecological crises.[5] Isn't it already an ecological crises when, because of the exhaustion of our soil and the use of artificial fertilizer and insecticides, our fruits and vegetables no longer contain the necessary concentration of vitamins, minerals, and trace elements, such as selenium and magnesium? These were still present fifty years ago, and it appears that we are genetically adapted to them.

"One of the most popular health measures today is the use of cereal juice."
(DONALD C. HEALTON, U.S. DEPARTMENT OF HEALTH AND WELFARE)

Even the scientific publications about barley grass in the USA during the 1950s reported that it contains all the nutrients that the human body needs (with the exception of vitamin D, which is produced in the skin). This combination of nutrients makes wheat grass and barley grass into "uniquely potent food."[6] Barley grass represents the best quality of organically cultivated green vegetable. In addition, this is a food that contains a concentrated form of beta carotene, calcium, chlorophyll, fiber, iron, and vitamin K. Furthermore, barley grass is a good source for proteins that are easily assimilated by the body, as well as vitamin C, vitamin B12, folic acid, vitamin B6 (pyridoxine), and many other trace elements.

It is important that the individual components in barley grass work together synergistically within the body. Ronald Seibold makes it clear that barley grass tablets are *not* multi-vitamin tablets. They are a concentrated combination of nutrients that can be found in all dark-green vegetables of a good quality. They work together for the good of the body as a whole. Cereal grasses like barley grass contain nutrients that support the functions of our interconnected vital systems and physiological processes.

If we think how outstandingly the various nutrients in barley grass work together in a synergetic manner, then we can only suggest that people look to such a food as this for support instead of to pills. In the following section, there are a few examples to illuminate the synergetic interaction of some of the nutrients in barley grass.[7]

Vitamin C is necessary for the absorption of calcium and iron. Iron is needed by the body to transform beta carotene into vitamin A. Calcium and pyridoxine (vitamin B6) help in the absorption of vitamin B12, which cannot be activated without folic acid. All of these nutrients are present in barley grass, together with many others that support similar functions.

Other examples of the synergistic interaction of nutrients are cited in Dr. Yoshihide Hagiwara's book *Green Barley Essence* (see Bibliography on page 146). Scientific studies carried out by Dr. Maurice E. Sill of Cornell University showed that the potassium and calcium level in the body fluids declines when there is a lack of magnesium. This even occurs when these minerals are ingested at an adequate level. When adequate magnesium absorption is ensured, the level of potassium and calcium rises automatically. Dr. Sill reports that magnesium is absolutely necessary for the correct mobilization of calcium in the bones and flesh, and also to keep potassium in the cells.[8] There is proof that stress, hard physical labor, sports, and working at night causes more sodium to be stored and potassium eliminated, which is expressed in constant fatigue. When its potassium content is too low, the body slows down its muscle movements and thought processes in order to prevent the further loss of potassium. We become tired and sleepy.[9] Barley grass is a very good source of potassium.

The German author Hans-Guenter Berner also criticizes the approach of using isolated "miracle" nutrients: He writes: "Our food is composed in a way that is much too clever for one single active ingredient to be the key to happiness."[10] There is apparently a great difference between which form and/or chemical compound of a vital substance is offered to the organism. "Intelligently developed vital-substance preparations are therefore oriented upon the blueprint of nature and not on the vitamin manufacturer's test tube."[11] Barley grass powder in its natural nutrient concentration and combination fulfills precisely this precondition of a food supplement created by nature.

Barley Grass or Wheat Grass?

Author Ronald L. Seibold basically equates barley grass juice and the products extracted from it with those of wheat grass. However, there are apparently ailments for which barley grass is preferable to wheat grass.

Wheat grass cures with seminars about nutrition with living foods are available in the institutes founded by Dr. Ann Wigmore in the USA, Puerto Rico, and Europe.[12]

Barley and Candida Patients

According to current estimates, 30 to 80 percent of all people living in the industrial nations suffer from mycosis (diseases caused by fungi). One of the leading types is infestation by Candida albicans. With its metabolic toxins, the fungi damages and weakens the organism. There is danger of the mycosis, which originally colonizes the intestines, spreading to the inner organs and the brain. Mycosis is nourished by all sweet, sugar-containing foods, which also includes the sweetish wheat grass. Candida patients should therefore avoid wheat grass juice and the powder extracted from it! The glucose it contains represents the ideal "food for intestinal fungi."

German author Halima Neumann has discovered that the health disorders of acidosis, cancer, and multiple sclerosis almost always are preceded by a fungal proliferation. She writes that after six months of a healing fast with wheat grass juice and green papaya juices, she could not cure her decades of suffering from candida; only when she changed over to the tart-bitter barley grass was it possible for her to achieve the desired normal state of not having a "distended belly."[13]

Candida patients should therefore prefer the tart-spicy barley grass and/or blue-green algae to the sweetish wheat grass. Dr. Yoshihide Hagiwara reports on numerous candida patients who were free of the fungi within a short time when they took the barley grass powder.

Nutritional Aspects of Barley Grass

Nutrient Concentration

Barley grass surpasses wheat grass in terms of the concentration level for most nutrients. This means that barley grass contains about twice as much of the easily assimilable calcium and twice as much potassium, which is important for the acid-alkali balance. At the same time, barley grass contains less than half the phosphorous of wheat grass, an element that is excessively present in our modern civilized diet. Experts such as Halima Neumann blame phosphorous for such problems as hyperactivity in children and sleep disorders in general. Furthermore, barley grass is also more abundant in chlorophyll and enzymes than wheat grass.

Tolerance

Fresh wheat grass juice is not tolerated by everyone; some people experience a feeling of nausea. On the other hand, barley grass juice, both the freshly squeezed and the powder that has been mixed with liquid, does not lead to stomach problems. This is probably because it neutralizes an excess of gastric acid since it is alkaline. According to Dr. Yoshihide Hagiwara, many wheat grass products are metabolized as an acid within the body. I would consider this a sign of denaturization in the production process (probably through temperatures that are too high) since fresh wheat grass is less alkaline than barley grass yet still is rich in alkaline.

Enzymes and Antioxidants

In contrast to wheat grass, barley grass contains the antioxidant enzyme, superoxide dismutase (SOD) to which I have devoted an entire chapter (see page 94), as well as the enzymes, fatty acid oxidase and transhydrogenase, which facilitate the breakdown of fats and the production of energy in the body. Individuals who have too little of these two enzymes frequently suffer from a storage of fat, weight problems, and an increased cholesterol level, with the danger of arteriosclerosis and thrombosis. Moreover, in comparison to wheat grass, barley grass contains catalase, an enzyme that activates the immune system in its battle against cancer cells.[14] Barley grass contains numerous antioxidants including the flavonoid, 2"-*O*-glycosyl-isovitexin (2"-*O*-GIV), which has been shown to be a more powerful antioxidant than beta-carotene, vitamin C, or vitamin E in preventing the oxidation of lipids. So far, 2"-*O*-GIV has not been found in any other vegetable or cereal grass examined except barley grass (also see page 85).

In contrast to wheat grass, dermatological studies by Dr. Tatsuo Muto, director of the *Muto Dermatologic Hospital* in Japan have determined that the enzyme complexes contained in barley grass are capable of healing pigmentation such as senile keratosis, melanosis, and skin impurities.[15] These research results have been confirmed by many people who drink barley grass juice or take the barley grass powder on a regular basis.

Bitter Constituents

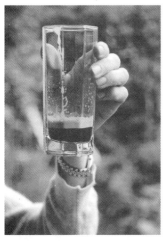

A further advantage of barley grass in comparison to wheat grass is the former substances' bitter constituents that primarily benefit the pancreas, the stomach, the liver, and the gallbladder. Bitter constituents are also abundantly contained in wild herbs and pot herbs.

The fresh juice of barley grass is mild and bitter at the same time. It can be creatively combined with almost any type of flavour. (Delicious recipes for it are on pages 116 ff.)

BARLEY GRASS FROM THE SPIRITUAL PERSPECTIVE

Jesus gathered his disciples under a tree and held a pot with wheat grass in his hands. "And the tender grass in the pot radiated life, just like the grass and the plants that cover the hills out to the distant fields and even beyond." Then Jesus gently stroked his hands over the grass, "as gently as if he were touching the head of a small child." At another point it says: "But of all things the most precious gift of your mother the earth is the grass beneath your feet, even the grass upon which you carelessly tread…Truly, I say unto you that the modest grass is more than food for the man and the animal." Jesus also spoke of the "secrets" hidden within the grass.

Jesus described the process of how the grain becomes cereal grass. The angel of the water and the angel of the air embrace the grain, and the angel of the sun awakens the life within it. Then the seedlings and roots are born within every seed-corn. And after the sun had risen four times, the grain turned into grass. "And truly I say unto you, there is no greater wonder than this."

Then Jesus explained to the disciples that the healing current of life, which produced the entire Creation, is visible and tangible in the grass: It is "…the meeting point of the earth mother and the heavenly father." The power of the sun is in the green of the grass and the other plants. Because the Son of Man was blinded by the bright light of the sun, "the angel of the sun transformed all of his life into green color, upon which the Son of Man looks upon the many different shades of green and finds strength and comfort." Then Jesus called the water in the blades the "water of life" and "the blood of the earth mother."

Jesus called each grain that grows up toward the heavens a "victory over death, where Satan rules, because life begins anew time and again." The angel of life flows through the blades of grass into the body of the Son of Light and shakes him with its strength.

"For the grass is life, and the Son of Light is life, and life flows between the Son of Light and the blades of grass and forms a bridge for the holy stream of light that gives life to the entire Creation."[16]

Developing Inner Qualities with Cereal Grass

Jesus invited his disciples to do a meditation with the cereal grass. They were asked to close their eyes and gently touch the grass. At first, the angel of **joy** filled their bodies with music. "When the Son of Man feels no joy in his heart, then he works for Satan…" The angel of **love** is also present in the blades of grass for "love is in life and great is the love that the Son of Light has been given through the tender blades of grass." When someone lovingly touches the blades of grass, they will return his love and accompany him to the streams of life. The angel of **wisdom** determines the communion of the Son of Light with the life stream through the tender blades of grass. **Peace** is the gift of the life stream to the Son of Light. "This is why you should always greet each other with "peace be with you," just as the grass greets your body with the kiss of peace."

Jesus also gave exact instructions for eating the grass: "Chew the blades well because the Son of Man has different teeth than the animals, and only when we chew well can the angel of water enter our blood and give us strength. O Sons of Light, eat from this perfect herb on the table of our earth mother so that your days on this earth may be long since this is pleasing to the eye of God." Every day, the disciples were to gather around the little earthen pots with the cereal grass that they had planted "with cheerful hearts together with the angels so that they accompany you on the healing stream of life…" The disciples were to convey a message of truth and light to the Sons of Man. "Loving means to constantly learn anew."

The Role of Barley Grass in the Bible

Dr. Mary Ruth Swope, a nutrition expert and author of *The Spiritual Roots of Barley*[17], apparently knows the Bible very well. Her basic assumption is that physical health and spiritual health are connected with each other on a very deep level and that barley grass plays a very special role in this process. As a teacher of nutrition over a time period of more than 50 years, she sees green barley as the most exciting ray of hope in terms of nutrition for overfed but undernourished

America. She recommends that every woman, man, and child take an adequate amount of dried green barley grass every day in order to improve the energy level and health on the cellular level.

Barley is a grass, and grasses are considered to be herbs in the botanic sense. The grasses are the most abundant family of green plants on the earth. Leviticus 23:10-12 speaks of a cereal offering, the first fruits. This refers to the leaves and fruits of barley, which, as the first ripe grains, are still given to God as an offering of thanks for Passover. Dr. Mary Ruth Swope goes as far as to say "what Jesus is for the spirit, barley is for our bodies."[18] All of the Biblical quotes that Dr. Mary Ruth Swope has collected cannot be listed here for reasons of space, but it is clear that she sees barley as a symbol for new life, completeness, and strength and as an important part of God's nutritional plan for us.[19] I sometimes find Dr. Mary Ruth Swope's interpretations a bit daring, but they are very inspiring and thought-provoking on the whole. Perhaps barley grass is a good opportunity for us to make our bodies into a "temple of God"!

Barley Connects Us with the Principle of "Light"

For the human being who is striving for higher ideals, barley is an important main food.

Some authors connect barley in particular with the principle of "light." This living, spiritual dimension that shines upon the grain gives human beings love, trust, meditation, the strength to give, and knowledge, among other qualities. In addition, barley promotes sensitivity, emotional stability, and pure, light-filled thought. On the physical level, according to some authors, it has a purifying and cleansing effect, as well as a strengthening effect on the muscular system.

In his classic on holistic nutrition Dr. Gabriel Cousens, American author and nutrition expert, discusses the question of which foods promote good health and spiritual growth. In addition to a portion of 35 to 40% fruit and the long-term conversion to 80 to 90% raw foods, he recommends eating more and more "biogenic" green plants like cereal grasses, sprouts, and young sunflowers on a regular basis since they are possibly the plants containing the most rejuvenating energy on the planet. Biogenic foods are qualitatively the best and highly life-giving and energy-providing. This type of food should be capable of producing a completely new organism.

According to Dr. Cousens—and in my experience as well—it is possible with such foods to maintain the experience of a loving state of oneness with God, increase the amount of energy required for awakening the kundalini energy, and intensify the experienced bliss of light and love, which includes the body, mind, and soul. Green juices support a meditative consciousness and make it easier to meditate. Dr. Cousens advises that we use green and fresh juices for this purpose, but he also says that this step exceeds what many people are willing to do in their lives.[20]

BARLEY GRASS FROM THE HISTORICAL PERSPECTIVE

Barley, the Oldest Grain in the World

Barley, the holy gift of the gods
(EGYPT)

Even in prehistoric times, grain was dried and roasted. Roasted barley from the Ice Age has been discovered, as well as from the Paleolithic era and the Neolithic period. The ancient Egyptians and Greeks also cultivated and roasted grain. Barley grows in Tibet at an elevation of up to 4400 meters, and it is even cultivated in the Sahara down to the region around the Equator.

Barley is the oldest sweet grass in the world and the oldest grain that has been cultivated. It comes from the Near East. With its straight, long leaves, it grows to a height of about one yard. Barley was cultivated even around 7000 years ago.

The North Dakota Barley Council has even traced the origins of barley back to 18,000 B.C.[21] Barley was the standard means of payment in Babylon. In addition to wheat, barley was the Egyptian's basic food 5000 years before Christ. According to legends, the Goddess Isis brought the people on the Nile grains of barley from Lebanon,[22] and it was even called "the holy gift of the gods" in ancient Egypt and Greece.

In ancient China, barley was considered to be a symbol of masculine potency because the ears of barley have "beards" (hair) and many seeds. Greek coins show the ears and stalks of barley. Roman gladiators were called "Hordearii" (barley-eaters) and went on strike when the barley rations were to be shortened during a war. In India, sacrifices were made to the Hindu god Indra for the good growth of the barley. Even thousands of years before Christ, the lake-dwellers of the Swiss Alps lived from barley. Christopher Columbus sailed under the royal flag of King Ferdinand and Queen Isabel of Spain to "El Mundo Nuevo" (the New World) and brought it barley. Later, American pioneers took the highly valued grain to the prairies of the West and the Pacific Coast.[23]

Basic Food of the Simple Folk

In the Middle Ages in Europe, the simple folk and farmers ate a heavy bread made of barley and rye. The more demanding wheat was first just cultivated here and there and reserved for the nobility. However, the more "fashionable" wheat soon supplanted barley. Today, there are still numerous varieties of barley. It is considered a nutritious food and is usually used in the form of flour, grits, flakes, and glazed grains. Its use as a drink dates back to prehistoric times when the barley grain was roasted, ground in a mortar, and mixed with water. Then it was fermented, which resulted in a foamy, wine-like drink that was the predecessor of beer. The Celts especially valued this drink. Today, barley is mainly cultivated as horse feed, as well as together with hops for the production of beer.

When fermented, the barley grain develops certain enzymes that cause malt to be created. In this form, starch can be absorbed particularly well by the body. Malt is given to patients, convalescents, small children, and older people as a restorative. Roasted malt as a coffee substitute has a good taste, is nourishing, and can be easily digested. Barley coffee made of roasted and ground barley grain is a well-known household remedy for gargling in the case of tonsillitis. Because of its gruel qualities, pearl barley is used in dietary cooking for calming a nervous stomach.

The barley sprout contains hordenin and an alkaloid that has a similar effect on the body as the hormone adrenaline, which increases blood pressure and stimulates heart activity. Barley has the effect of raising blood pressure when it is too low and balances high blood pressures, meaning that it can regulate the heart. It has a calming, sedative effect and is also taken against diarrhea. "Barley water," which is a decoction from peeled barley grain, rightfully has the reputation of being a mild tonic. In external applications, especially as a warm compress, it has a soothing and calming effect.

Without spelt as a whole grain or even as whole-grain flour, barley still has a surprising number of nutrients to offer. The healthiest and most nutritious form is the barley grain that is sprouted.

A Familiar Healing Remedy in Biblical Times

However, even in comparison to the barley grain, barley grass is a much more powerful and potent healing food. The Essenes of Jesus' time were probably not only familiar with wheat grass as a healing remedy and food, but also barley grass. According to the Book of Daniel in the Old Testament, King Nebuchadnezzar (630 to 562 B.C.) just lived from grass for seven years. Afterward, he claimed that he could once again think clearly and rule his kingdom.

We know that the ancient cultures of the Orient and Middle East ate the young grasses of wheat and barley.[24] The Egyptians of antiquity are also said to already have been familiar with barley grass and alfalfa as a food supplement and restorative. The Indians of North America used barley grass both externally and internally for healing purposes.[25] The Celtic Druids in Scotland, Ireland, and northern France also used barley grass juice, in addition to wheat grass juice, to heal wounds and as a "magic po-tion" for their own tribes in mili-tary campaigns.[26] Cereal grasses also supposedly played a role for the Indian tribes in Central America as a wound-healing rem-edy; furthermore, they were a blood-purifying and restorative remedy in China under the em-perors of the Ming Dynasty dur-ing the Middle Ages.

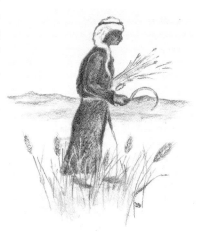

Phaeton—Awakening from Time

Transformation occurs
What is concealed
Reaches for you,
Power wants to hide itself
From the changes.
The fire bursts you,
The day glistens on you,
The light releases you.

Humus is created,
Illuminates your new path.
The Goddess of Darkness gives birth,
Frees her children,
Collects upon the earth
What is hers,
Takes new paths,
Conceals new power
In the dawning of a new morning.

The earth was once burned
By the fall of the light
Tenderness and love
Will become new.
The grass grows again,
Rings in a new age,
Triumphs
In heaven
As on earth.

MONIKA HELMKE-HAUSEN

CEREAL GRASSES FROM THE SCIENTIFIC PERSPECTIVE

One of the first people in modern times to discover the healing power of barley grass and scientifically study it was the physician Dr. Charles F. Schnabel from the Kansas City Rockhurst College in Kansas City, in 1928. He noticed that hens fed with the blood-forming plant material in the form of cereal grass laid many more eggs and lived much longer than those fed with normal chicken feed. By simply increasing the supplementary feeding with cereal grasses by ten percent, the production of eggs in winter increased by 38 to 94 percent! Not only were there more eggs laid but the eggs also had considerably harder shells, from which much healthier chicks developed than from the eggs of normally fed hens. Dr. Charles F. Schnabel wrote that even a child could recognize the blossoming health of the grass-fed hens.[27]

While I was writing these lines, I stayed at an organic finca on the Canary island of La Palma. I began feeding barley grass and alfalfa sprouts to the eight hens there; the result was that they doubled their production of eggs within three days!

Encouraged by these experiences, Dr. Charles Schnabel made a dried extract from cereal grasses and gave it to the seven members of his family. *The Buffalo Courier Express* of June 1, 1942 reported on Dr. Charles Schnabel, writing that none of his children had ever been seriously ill or had bad teeth. Dr. Charles Schnabel, greatly ahead of his time, then developed a nutritional plan for the hungering peoples of the world on the basis of a high-grade protein food supplement from cereal grasses. Since the beginning of the 1930s, barley grass powder has been available in the USA as the "first multivitamin pill in the world."

Barley Grass for Preventing Miscarriages

In the middle of the 1930s, Dr. George Kohler at the University of Wisconsin discovered that the higher nutritional value of milk in summer came from the grass that the cows ate in the spring and summer. He then intensively researched this grass-juice factor. In 1940,

Dr. George Kohler discovered that the young cereal grass fed to the dairy cows resulted in a much higher milk output. As a result, a physician in Kansas City gave dried cereal grass to pregnant women in danger of miscarriage with great success. Since the 1930s, dried cereal grass has been available in the USA as a food supplement.

Dr. Ann Wigmore Rang in a Renaissance of Cereal Juices

Cereal grass juices were rediscovered during the 1960s and 1970s in the USA during the course of growing environmental and health consciousness. Dr. Ann Wigmore, who had become seriously ill during the middle years of her life and then remembered that her grandmother had healed the wounds of soldiers in the First World War with squeezed grain juice, made a great contribution to this Renaissance. (More about Dr. Ann Wigmore in the section starting on page 44.) In 1968, she established the Hippocrates Health Institute in Boston, famous in health circles in the USA, where she healed patients who orthodox medicine had given up on as incurably ill through grass juices, other green foods, sprouts, and raw foods.

Probably the most famous patient, who was able to leave Dr. Ann Wigmore's institute with his illness cured in 1969, was Viktoras Kulvinskas.*

Dr. Yoshihide Hagiwara Discovered
"the Most Perfect Food in the World"

At about the same time that Dr. Ann Wigmore worked in Boston, the scientist Dr. Yoshihide Hagiwara became involved with the health advantages of cereal grasses on the other side of the globe. He began to search for the healthiest food in the world. Similar to Dr. Charles Schnabel about fifty years earlier, he came to the conclusion that the leaves of the cereal grasses provide the nearest thing this planet offers to the perfect food. Of all the foods that he had tested, he discovered that the young leaves of barley and certain other types of cereal grasses had the most remarkable amounts of active components.[28]

---

* His book, *Survival into the 21ˢᵗ Century,* (see Bibliography on page 146) became a classic in the field of natural nutrition. To this day, he is still active holding lectures, seminars, and writing books to promote more green foods and health consciousness.

Dr. Yoshihide Hagiwara decided upon barley grass as the ideal food supplement for human beings for a variety of reasons. For example, barley sprouts germinated more quickly at a temperature of less than 15 degrees C, a temperature at which the troublesome mold fungi and bacteria cannot exist. Furthermore, barley grass fulfills the following criteria: the greatest nutrient quality, best harvesting conditions, and a good taste. He developed an extract from barley grass with a small amount of maltodextrin, and brown rice as an additional ingredient: Green Magma or Green Barley Essence—and called it the ideal "fast food" for modern people.

The "Green Revolution" Hasn't Even Started Yet

Today, the health value of cereal grasses for human nutrition is experiential knowledge that has not only been confirmed many thousands of times but has also been confirmed by extensive clinical studies and laboratory experiments, primarily since the end of the 1960s in the USA and Japan. According to Ronald L. Seibold, these two movements, together with an increased availability of cereal grass that has been cultivated in America and prepared in a way that protects the nutrients, are responsible for a renaissance in the use of cereal grasses as food for human beings. In the USA, some vegetarian restaurants and natural food stores offer freshly squeezed barley grass or wheat grass juice and tablets made of cereal grasses.

Dr. Ann Wigmore:
The Cereal Juice Pioneer

She Healed Seriously Ill Patients with Barley Grass Juice

Dr. Ann Wigmore originally came from Lithuania. She observed how her grandmother healed soldiers who had been injured in the First World War with the wheat grass and barley grass juice that she gave her patients to drink and applied to their wounds. Ann Wigmore, who had immigrated to the USA in the meantime, became seriously ill with colitis (inflammation of the large intestine). At that point, she remembered her grandmother's art of healing and began to chew on the wheat grass and barley grass that grew near her home. After a short time, she was not only healed of her illness but her hair—which had already turned white—returned to its original brown color.

To make things more convenient for herself, Ann Wigmore began to squeeze the juice and drink it. After she had experienced such success with herself, she began to feed her dogs and cats green juice additives from wheat grass and barley grass. In one of the many tele-

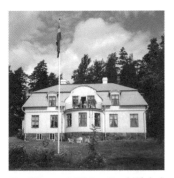

Dr. Wigmore's Living Food Global Center in Skeppsgården, Sweden, which is where she treated people with grass juices and raw foods rich in enzymes.

phone conversations we had with each other, Ann Wigmore said that they also became much more active and peppy, and made a rejuvenated and energetically charged impression, as if they had been transformed.

The reputation of her "magic health elixir" quickly spread around her neighborhood and she began to provide many of her sick neighbors and friends with the green juices. The success even astonished her: Many people were able to leave their beds for the first time in years, and some of them could even go back to work as if nothing had happened! She could hardly believe this miracle.

In 1968, Dr. Wigmore established the Hippocrates Health Institute in Boston where she primarily treated people with degenerative diseases who could expect little help from orthodox medicine. Above all, the treatment consisted of wheat grass juice, barley grass juice, and raw foods rich in enzymes. Since she was not a physician (she had her PhD), many of her numerous seminar-participants lived for free as her "guests" in her institute. Private donations were secretly and unofficially given to her in envelopes since she was not officially permitted to accept any proceeds from her work.[29]

Cereal Grasses Help Against Almost All Health Disorders, Even Cancer

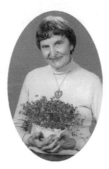

Dr. Ann Wigmore, the cereal grass juice pioneer, was both a wonderful woman and a pioneer

Dr. Ann Wigmore, who was in her Eighties, tragically died a few years ago in a fire in her laboratory. She was proud that she had taken care of many people whom the physicians had given up on because they no longer responded to the conventional medical treatments after surgical operations, radiation, and/or chemotherapy. Many people reported that the physicians had sent them to Dr. Ann Wigmore with these words: "If we now hand you over to this woman, at least you will die because of quackery and not through our hands or our methods." Many patients who sometimes couldn't even walk and had to be carried to her on a stretcher, not only became healthy but felt even better than before and spread the good news of their recovery.

Dr. Ann Wigmore believed that barley grass juice and wheat grass juice were a healing remedy for almost every disease. She even achieved breathtaking results with alcoholics, drug addicts, young people addicted to sugar, people with states of exhaustion, infections, and the widespread malnutrition. Her student Viktoras Kulvinskas and the Japanese pharmacist Dr. Yoshihide Hagiwara also worked very successfully with green juices, but Dr. Ann Wigmore was unique in her pioneer achievements as a researcher on the many healing effects of wheat grass juice and barley grass juice for numerous health disorders. Time and again, she said that she had even been able to heal the supposedly "incurable!"

At Eighty, as Fit and Vital as a 35-Year Old

I was able to speak to Dr. Ann Wigmore on the phone a number of times and am acquainted with several people who personally knew Dr. Ann Wigmore. All of them report that although she was over eighty years old, she had the charisma and vitality of a woman in her mid-thirties up to the end. Slim and slender like a young deer, she jumped back and forth between her sprouting containers and tablets with wheat grass. These were her standard equipment, without which she never traveled. She also always had a wheat grass juicer with her that she used to extract the juice from her 5-day wheat and her barley in hotel rooms. When asked if all of this didn't create a lot of work for her, she replied that it did, but was worth the effort. She was an eighty-year-old grandmother with the physical fitness and energy of a thirty-five-year-old.

It is possible to visit the seminars at the Ann Wigmore Center in the USA in West Palm Beach, Florida and order her books there. [30+12]

People who have been healed by Dr. Ann Wigmore through her grass juice therapy thank her not only for their lives but also for a quality of life that they had never considered to be possible for themselves. Eydie Mae Hunsberger, a former cancer patient: "Ann's juice therapy gave me back *my life*! This is a renewal of life that I had never dreamed of in the miserable state of health in which I found myself back then!"[31] (Dr. Ann Wigmore has written many books, see Bibliography on page 147 ff.)

Dr. Yoshihide Hagiwara:
The Discoverer of Barley Grass

"Let your food be your medicine"
(HIPPOCRATES)

Dr. Yoshihide Hagiwara was born in 1925 in Oita, Japan. After the Second World War, he lived in Hiroshima and was confronted with the disastrous effects of the radiation there. In 1949, he completed his university studies with a degree in pharmacology and opened the *Dr. Hagiwara Pharmacy* in Osaka. He devoted a great deal of his leisure time to the research of new medications. After the development of several very successful drug preparations, he established one of the largest pharmaceutical businesses in Japan. In 1960, he became a general practitioner.

As a result of his own long ordeal, Dr. Yoshihide Hagiwara was faced with the fact that many chemical preparations only suppress the symptoms of an illness but cannot truly heal diseases. In the

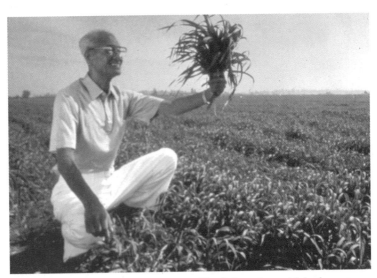

Dr. Yoshihide Hagiwara first healed himself and then others with barley grass juice—he is one of the people who advanced the scientific studies of barley grass juice in an incomparable manner. The photo shows him at one of his plantations.

Green Barley Essence, the Ideal "Fast Food," (see Bibliography on page 146 ff.) he describes how he poisoned himself with organic mercury while developing his own new medication: He and his staff developed red spots on the nose and the skin peeled while they were attempting to create a medicine that helps against skin problems. Dr. Yoshihide Hagiwara's teeth fell out and his hair turned gray—but he was only 38 years old! He noticed how his mental and physical powers were quickly disappearing. His attempts to become fit through vitamin tablets and hormone shots were unsuccessful. Frustrated, he recognized that the vitamin tablets and medications he had developed to combat states of exhaustion were apparently useless.

He Neglected His Own Health While He Researched the Health of Others

To make matters worse, Dr. Yoshihide Hagiwara had become accustomed to a very unhealthy diet and lifestyle. Because of the excessive amount of work he had to do, he only allowed himself three hours of sleep a day and his meals usually consisted of hamburgers or rice with curry. For ten years, he ate curry and rice at lunch and a hamburger-steak in the late evening, accompanied by a soft drink: He claims he was simply too busy to take the time for preparing a more healthy meal. It's no wonder that his physical and mental performance was deteriorating. Dr. Yoshihide Hagiwara recognized that although he was dedicating his life to the idea of contributing to the health of humanity, he had irresponsibly neglected his own health in the process. This perception became the turning point of his life.

Dr. Yoshihide Hagiwara began to intensively study Chinese herb preparations. Even as a child, the traditional Japanese diet with many vegetables, potatoes, soy beans, and millet gruel had saved him by healing his severe tuberculosis. He wasn't able to go to school for an entire year because of his disease! His research confirmed that the power of green leaves as a food had formed the source for life and the well-being of the human body—up until the 20th century. He believes that the continuous decrease of natural green power in the human diet is the most serious threat to our health, more than any other factor.

Cereal Grasses,
the Ideal Food for Human Beings

How did Dr. Yoshihide Hagiwara come up with the idea that cereal grasses are the ideal food for human beings? At the time that he was working with the green vegetable juices and analyzing their contents, he visited a farmer on the Chita Peninsula in the southwest of Japan. It was summer, but he couldn't find any of the rice plants that normally grow everywhere in Japan during this season. Instead, he saw Italian rye grass, rye, and large areas of dark-green oats. Dr. Yoshihide Hagiwara knew that the sale of rice brought about $1,600 per hectare, while only $120 was paid for green rye leaves. So he naturally asked the farmer why he was wasting his land on unprofitable grain. The farmer's answer was that he could achieve an increased yield of $4,900 a year through his cows when they were fed the rye leaves instead of hay or pasture grass. He added that the period in which a cow gave milk was extended by five to six years through this feed. Dr. Yoshihide Hagiwara was astonished to learn in this way of the ability the green cereal grasses have for creating so much vitality and energy.

The study of about 200 chlorophyll-containing plants for nutrient concentration and optimal nutrient composition led Dr. Yoshihide Hagiwara to green barley grass. Of all the plants that he tested, the young shoots of barley had the most remarkable amounts of active components. Barley grass is rich in minerals and vitamins, contains twice as much high-quality protein as wheat-grain, as well as much cellulose and few calories. The result of his efforts was green barley essence, which is available in stores as a product called Green Magma. This is a

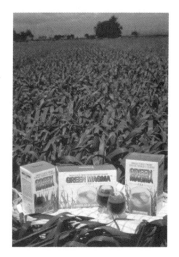

Dr. Yoshihide Hagiwara describes his extract from barley grass juice as having a pleasant mild taste like green tea with fresh peas or like that of tender spinach.

gently dried and pulverized juice of barley grass, which has been harvested and processed at the time of the most optimal nutrient concentration.

Dr. Yoshihide Hagiwara was also convinced by the taste: His barley grass juice tastes pleasantly like green tea with fresh peas or its taste is reminiscent of tender spinach. In addition, his product is perfect for our age—mixing the juice just takes a few seconds—and the powder can be stored for an almost unlimited time.

Dr. Yoshihide Hagiwara Showered with Awards

With his product, Dr. Yoshihide Hagiwara won the Pharmaceutical Meritorious Service Award in 1982; in 1987, he won the prize from the General Director of the Science and Technology Agency, established by the Japanese Ministry for Science and Technology, for his method of making powder from the young barley plants. Today, Dr. Yoshihide Hagiwara is the acting director of the Japan Kanpo Shoyaku Manufacturers Association, a group that is involved with Chinese herbs, and director of the non-profit association Japan Health Food Association. In 1992, Dr. Yoshihide Hagiwara spent one year as a guest professor at the University of California in Davis, California. In 1994, he received an additional award, the Drug and Medical Meritorious Service Award (from the Japanese Ministry for Science and Technology) for the development of unique techniques for extracting and stabilizing vitamins, minerals, and living enzymes for food in powder form. In 1995, Dr. Yoshihide Hagiwara was honored with a prize from the Brazilian government for the improvement in the health of the world's people. In 1990, Dr. Yoshihide Hagiwara opened an additional production site for Green Magma in Oxnard, California.

Medicine Should Protect Humanity from Disease

Dr. Yoshihide Hagiwara's motto is that the actual goal of medicine should be to protect humanity against disease and promote physical and mental fitness. He considers the discovery of such a large amount of active, health-promoting substances in young barley leaves to be "a revelation from heaven." Dr. Yoshihide Hagiwara has established a non-profit foundation, the Association of Green and Health, as well as the private research institute that he founded in 1970, the Hagiwara Institute of Health, in Kasai, Japan where about twenty researchers work. Many internationally renowned scientists like Dr. Mendelssohn from the Cancer Center of the University of San Diego have already visited this institute. Scientists from all over the world are welcomed by Dr. Yoshihide Hagiwara to learn about the work of his institute and present suggestions.[32]

Dr. Mary Ruth Swope: Competent Barley Grass Enthusiast

Dr. Mary Ruth Swope is a best-selling author. Her book, *Green Leaves of Barley* (see Bibliography on page 147 ff.), has sold several hundred thousand copies alone. For more than fifty years, she has been active in the field of nutritional counseling and education. She received her Ph.D. at Columbia University in New York City. She earned her other university degrees in South Carolina, graduating in the field of food and nutrition from the University of North Carolina. For more than twenty years, she taught as a dean at the School for Home Economics of the Eastern Illinois University in Charleston, Illinois.

Both Dr. Mary Ruth Swope's books, *Green Leaves of Barley* and *The Spiritual Roots of Barley* are very informative. She wrote the first book together with Dr. David A. Darbro, a physician and ambassador of the American Board of Chelation Therapy. He has become a familiar figure in the USA through his television appearances and health seminars. I think the *Green Leaves of Barley* book is the most well-founded book about barley grass and the important role of proper nutrition for our health, written in a very engaging manner. She makes no secret of her enthusiasm about the dried juice of young barley grass and a healthy diet with much "living," enzyme-rich plant food. According to Dr. Mary Ruth Swope, cells that have been strengthened by good food will travel a long distance by giving us an immune system that resists the diseases of this modern age, which have become so prevalent in our society.

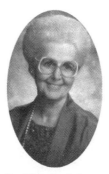

Dr. Mary Ruth Swope

An Advocate of Holistic, Gentle Medicine

How did Dr. Mary Ruth Swope, who looks so friendly as she smiles radiantly on the cover of her main work, discover the important significance of nutrition for our health? In contrast to Dr. Ann Wigmore and Dr. Yoshihide Hagiwara, it was not her own personal suffering but the illness of a family member that caused her to feel helpless with her conventional medical approach. Although she had previously laughed at naturopathic doctors as "quacks," she was forced to place a beloved family member in the hands of such a "quack." And his therapy worked!

Even before this time, she had become painfully aware that her patients never became truly healthy. She had to come to terms with having to keep diseases at an acceptable level: and this was a shock for her. She gradually began to think about this and question her previous kind of knowledge until she herself became an advocate of holistic, gentle medicine.

Dr. Mary Ruth Swope confronted her readers with appalling figures about the state of health of the American people, although the situation was not much better anywhere else. Seventy percent of deaths in the USA can be attributed to diseases that are related to dietary habits. The USA holds the world record for osteoporosis patients: about one-third of the American women suffer from it after menopause, and this health disorder is also affecting young women and men for the first time in the history of the USA. From 1960 to 1986, the number of deaths because of cancer increased by 223%, and the American Institute of Cancer Research estimates that 60% of these cases can be traced to improper nutrition. Dr. Mary Ruth Swope sees a relationship between the consumption of soft drinks and the consumption of meat and fish.

Barley Grass for Radiant Health

Many of the best-educated physicians believe that the medications currently prescribed are full of side effects and are useless, if not lethal (deadly) for sick people, according to Dr. Mary Ruth Swope. In contrast to this, she repeatedly emphasizes that healthy foods do not have any life-threatening accompanying symptoms but have radiant health as their only side-effect. Her basic statement is that if Americans want to be healed from cancer, heart disease, arthritis, diabetes, excess weight and an entire long list of debilitating conditions, they must find unconventional methods of healing that include the food and healing remedies provided by nature as their main components.

Spray-dried barley grass juice are an excellent example of a natural food when they are cultivated without chemical fertilizers and pesticides and not preserved with heat or freezing. Today, the greater portion of the foods that we can buy in the supermarket are "dead." Although they may taste good, they cannot provide the cells with the nutrients they need to create and maintain a healthy body. We must change the conditions for chronic diseases for which there is no medical healing and take personal responsibility for preventing these diseases.

BARLEY GRASS PRODUCTS

Organically Grown Barley Grass

Barley grass has been a "hit" among food supplements in the USA and Japan for decades. One of the barley grass products developed by Dr. Yoshihide Hagiwara is the best-selling food supplement in Japan.

Barley grass is a natural, highly concentrated food supplement: 100 g provide the nutritional value of four pounds of the best organic vegetables! A heaping teaspoon of Green Magna has the same nutritional value as two to three portions of raw, organically grown vegetables.

Hardly anyone really follows the cancer research institutes' recommendation that we should eat five to seven servings of fruit and vegetables every day. That is why anyone who would like to achieve good health or stay healthy should drink barley grass juice several times a day.

Even if you don't have the time or don't want to grow barley grass on your windowsill or in the garden, you can still take advantage of this valuable food. Natural food stores, health food stores, and mail-order companies have quite a large selection of barley grass extracts in powder form. These can be used to make barley grass juice by stirring one to two teaspoons of the green powder into a glass with non-carbonated water or fruit and vegetable juices that are low in acids (see the recipe section of this book on page 116 ff. for ideas). This barley grass is grown without the use of herbicides and pesticides on large farms, in the USA, Australia, Japan, and also in other countries.

Winter barley grass even grows well in colder climates. Sowed in the autumn, the barley requires about 200 days to reach the optimal nutrient concentration. At the stage of the highest nutritional content, it is gently processed at temperatures below 50 degrees C in order to preserve as many of the enzymes and other nutrients as possible.

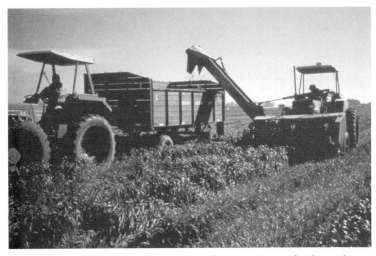

The organic cultivation on large farms uses efficient equipment for the gentle harvest of the barley grass

Within two to three hours after the harvest, the barley grass has already been processed and the washing procedure, the extraction of the juice, and the spray-drying process take place at body temperature, which gently protects the enzymes. The cellulose is returned to the barley grass fields as a natural fertilizer.

The instant juice powder created in this manner, Green Magma from American and Japanese organic cultivation, can be easily dissolved and has a pleasant sweet taste. It also contains some maltodextrin and brown rice. Maltodextrin is a natural, complex carbohydrate that coats the enzymes so that they cannot react with each other but only become active when dissolved in water. This product is also suitable for diabetics and does not contain gluten, which can trigger allergies. The brown rice increases its level of vitamin B and holds the fine green powder together. Almost all of the fibrous substances are removed from the Green Magma in order to make the barley grass juice easier to digest and assimilate so that the body can

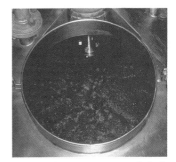

This is a large container with fresh barley grass juice

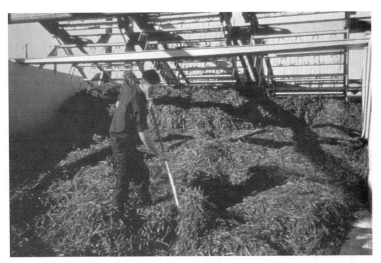

The cut barley is processed immediately after it is harvested

absorb the nutrients within twenty minutes. According to information from the manufacturer, the human body is not capable of completely digesting the roughage in barley grass or the nutrients that this roughage contains within it.

However, the important mineral potassium, which is vital for the muscles, nerves, metabolism, and our acid-alkaline balance, is primarily found in these fibrous materials, according to nutrition experts. Anyone who is too acidic—see part on acidosis in this book on page 130 ff.—should therefore perhaps either use other barley grass products or increase the dosage of Green Magma.

Since this product is free of roughage, it is especially well suited for barley grass fasting treatments since it is gentle to the intestines in an optimal manner. Green Magma is also available in tablet form. It can also be purchased as a supplement to cat food and dog food.

Barley Grass in Lozenge Form

Barley grass powder is available in tablet form from various makers. This is usually pressed barley grass powder. Let the tablets dissolve slowly in your mouth or swallow them and drink liquids with them, if possible. The taste is usually slightly bitter and therefore some people may need to get used to it.

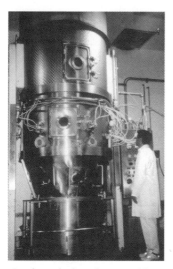

Gentle methods make it possible to process barley grass powder or pressed tablets while protecting of as much of the vital-substance concentration as possible.

Particularly bitter components, as they are also found in many pot herbs and wild herbs in particular, are hardly to be found in our modern-day diets. Yet, they are very important for the optimal functioning of the stomach, liver, and gallbladder.

If you can't get used to the taste, you can also take coated barley grass extract tablets.

Especially children, who frequently will not accept something that tastes bitter, will enjoy these tablets or Green Magma, which does not taste bitter, as the healthy alternative. My son always has a jar of these barley grass tablets in his schoolbag and uses them as an energy-providing snack at recess or as brain food before classroom tests. Because barley grass contains glutamine acid and the antioxidant enzyme, SOD it is an ideal food for supporting mental activity.

Barley grass is also used in combination with other supplements in order to enhance the synergy of beneficial effects that occur with a variety of different phytochemicals acting together. For instance, the company, Wakunaga of America, manufactures a supplement that contains a combination of barley grass, blue-green algae and garlic. They claim that this combination produces beneficial effects greater than if each ingredient was taken separately.

Freshly Squeezed Juice
or Barley Grass Juice from Powder?

What should we give preference to: the freshly squeezed barley grass juice that we grow ourselves or grass juice made from extracted barley grass powder? There are various opinions on this topic. Like many other people, I use both the freshly squeezed barley grass juice *and* the instant juice powder with great success. Dr. Ann Wigmore recommends juicing the fresh cereal grasses since she believes that the vital force is greater in the fresh juices than in the dried: Dried products may be a good source of nutrients, but they contain little of the vital force (the energy from the enzymes) that we find in the fresh grass juices.

On the other hand, the producers of barley grass powder and tablets point out that only at the optimal time of maturity—when the nutrient concentration is the greatest—is the simple sugar in the grass converted into the complex carbohydrates that are valuable for our health. This time of the greatest nutrient concentration, the jointing stage that occurs just before the stalk pushes up out of the grass, cannot be achieved by growing the grass on the windowsill. Grain that is grown indoors will fail to produce a seed head.

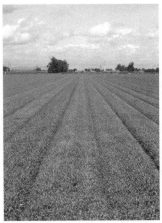

The nutrient concentration of barley grass is ultimately also dependent upon the quality of the soil

Barley Grass Grows Best on "Untouched" Soil

Producers of barley grass products including Pines International, Wakunaga of America (Kyo-Green), Green Foods Corporation (Green Magma) and some others have their own patented production methods. The result is that there is a minimum loss of vitamins and enzymes and their products are raw-food quality, meaning that these are still "living" products.

The reports on healing that Dr. Yoshihide Hagiwara collected through the decades and the scientific studies speak for the high quality of enzyme-active barley grass extract.

Another decisive factor for the quality of the product is the nutrient concentration of the soil. Dr. Yoshihide Hagiwara established his American branch only after doing numerous soil analyses in an area with mineral-rich soil—Oxnard, California. The suppliers of barley grass products from organically grown barley in Australia, which are offered under the label of *Green Barley*, point out the high quality of their mineral-rich "untouched" soil.

As Ronald L. Seibold writes in his book *Cereal Grass, What's In It for You,* that homegrown cereal grass apparently has powerful cleansing qualities and is therefore very successfully used as therapy for chronic health disorders. He believes that its value appears to be more in its cleansing and medical effect than the fact that it is a green vegetable food. However, the cleansing and medical effects of various barley grass extracts are also well documented.

For our bodies, we need powerful cleansing and purifying remedies, as well as an optimal supply of nutrients. And this is not just on an occasional basis, but several times every day, if possible. On my windowsill and in the garden during the summer, I grow barley grass that I chew or juice and mix my barley grass drink from powder at least three times a day. When I travel, I always have barley grass tablets with me as a quick pick-me-up. They also help neutralize the exhaust from the cars in traffic and immediately give me the energy I need. I invite the readers to try out both possibilities and profit from both of them! If you don't have much time or don't feel like growing the barley grass yourself, the barley grass products give you the opportunity of instantly doing something profound for your health, mental alertness, and good mood.

Barley Grass Cultivation

Growing Barley Grass at Home: Easier Than You Think!

It is very easy to grow your own barley or wheat grass at home. To do this, you will need germinable seeds from the health food store or natural food store.

The best place to germinate the grain is not a sprouting container since poor ventilation can be a problem but one-quart pickle jars. In addition, you will need gauze (a wide-meshed, porous cotton material), and a preserving ring to hold it in place. For each jar, use about four heaping tablespoons of grain. Cover the grain with water and let it soak for 12 hours, overnight, for example. The next morning, rinse the grain well under flowing water. Pour off the old water, fill it with fresh water, and drain the water off. Then place the jar at an angle facing the window, whereby the end of the jar should be placed on a pastry board. This provides good ventilation for the grain. Repeat this process twice a day, in the morning and the evening.

After two to three days, depending on the temperature, the grain will sprout and the tender roots become visible. Now the grain is ready for planting. Rinse the grain one more time and place the seeds closely together—but not on top of each other—on a tablet, bowl, baking tin, or something similar that has been filled at least five centimeters (two inches) high with organic soil (garden store) or compost soil. Press the sprouted grain lightly into the soil. Now spray everything with water (plant or laundry sprayer).

Keep the grain in the dark for three to five days by covering it with

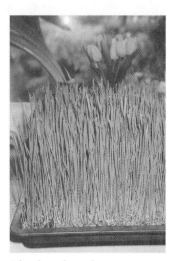

The photo shows the green grass at the length that is optimal for a harvest at home

something like a baking tin so that the roots can develop well and strong plants can grow from them. Then expose the little barley plants to the sunlight. The ideal place for this would be the windowsill of a window facing south so that the chlorophyll can be formed. During the vegetation period, barley grass can also be grown in the garden or in flower boxes on the balcony. Spray the seedlings with water once or twice a day to keep them moist. When they have grown into grass, you can water them carefully with the sprinkling can. However, too much water can lead to the formation of mold.

When properly planted and cared for, two sprouting beds the size of a baking tin yield about two pounds of grass, from which 300 g of juice can be extracted. In order to extract this amount of juice, two beds must be planted every two days. The harvest begins between the seventh and the fourteenth day, when the blades have reached a height of three to four inches.

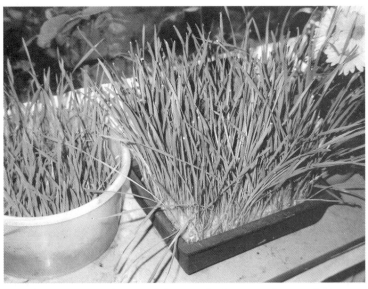

Only the simplest utensils are needed to grow barley grass at home—whether in the garden or on the window sill during the colder seasons, the grass always thrives and grows quickly.

Frequent Errors

When good-quality grain only yields a meager harvest, this may be because they were soaked for too long. In summer, the grain should be soaked for 12 hours at most; in the winter, they can be soaked for up to 24 hours. If the juice tastes bitter or flat, the soil is poor in quality and it must be replaced with better soil. If you add some seaweed (natural food store), kelp from sea algae (health food store), the juice will become even richer in minerals and taste sweeter.

If the grass has too little light and sunshine, it will become dry and pale. If it is growing in a dark room, you can use a 40-watt infrared bulb. If the soil is too loamy, you should mix some sand in with it so that the grass can develop well. Earthworms make the soil more porous and provide it with oxygen.

If the soil molds, the grass has received too much moisture and/or has been planted too densely. The soil should be kept moist, but not wet, and it also shouldn't be allowed to dry out.

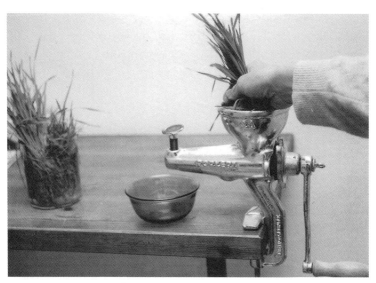

The juice can be extracted quickly and gently with a hand-operated cereal grass juicer

Juice Extraction: By Chewing or Using a Juicer

When the cereal grass blades have grown to be about three to four inches, they have received a maximum of enzymes and nutrients at this point. Now you can "harvest" them by simply cutting them just above the roots with scissors or a sharp knife. I always cut only as much as I need. The cut grass will keep in the refrigerator when placed in a closed jar. In the meantime, the turf will grow a second harvest. However, this has only half of the healing power and nutrient concentration as the first harvest.

You can also put small bushels of the cereal grass in your mouth, chew it thoroughly, and just swallow the juice. Spit out the cellulose that remains after chewing the grass and swallowing the juice. This is the simplest and most natural way to extract the juice. Especially when I'm driving the car, I always take along a little plastic bag with barley grass or wheat grass blades. This is the ideal snack for immediately replacing the energy I've used.

Those who would like a somewhat more "respectable" method can purchase a hand-operated or electrical cereal grass juicer. I only use a juicer when I plan to make larger amounts of juice for guests because cleaning the machine for just one grass juice meal is too much work for me. Viktoras Kulvinskas is critical of the normal electrically operated juicers and says that the juice oxidizes and consequently loses its nutrients. He therefore recommends the use of a normal grain mill: use a cloth as a sieve for the finely ground mass, pressing on it with a spoon.[33] I have had good experiences in making barley grass juice with the electrical juicers. These juicers are very well suited for making fresh fruit and vegetable juices.

The Remaining Fibrous Material for Healing Purposes

The remaining fibrous material can be used in healing and regenerating compresses for all types of skin disorders and wounds, or as suppositories against hemorrhoids. As first aid for injuries, chew the barley grass or wheat grass and place the juicy fibers on the afflicted area.

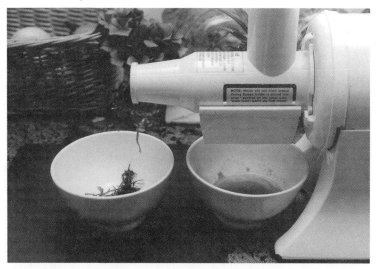

An electrical juicer can be used to make juice more conveniently and quickly. This is especially useful in large operations like sanatoriums and healing centers.

It is best to drink the barley grass juice immediately (and mix it well with your saliva) because it loses a considerable amount of its healing effect through oxidation after just ten minutes. Sealed tightly and kept in the refrigerator, the juice only has a therapeutic value for about twelve hours.

Never drink more than four ounces of juice extract at once. Always dilute it with eight ounces of water because the toxins and waste substances may reach the bloodstream too quickly and lead to nausea and dizziness when the dosage is too high.

Chewing

I prefer to chew the grass because this method optimally preserves the nutrients and extraction with a wheat grass juicer or spinach grinder is a bit too time-consuming! To do this, chew the spicy, sweetish grass until the fibrous material becomes tasteless.

Don't swallow the fibrous material because it could become entangled in the intestinal villi. Between mouthfuls, sip four to eight ounces of water. This chewing also activates the brain circulation, as well as strengthening the gums and healing gum bleeding and paradontosis.

Even the Sod Is Useful: Wonderful Compost

The cut sod can be quickly transformed into wonderful compost. A plastic bucket with a lid can be used as a composter. Drill ventilation holes into the four outer walls at a distance of two inches apart. The container can be placed in the garden or on the balcony: The rotting process takes place without any bad smells. Fill the sides of the bucket with cereal grass sod and place soil with earthworms from finished compost in the center. After about two months, you will have a wonderful fertile flower and garden soil that you can also use for new indoor grain fields.

You can naturally cultivate barley grass and wheat grass outdoors in the summer (and other seasons in warmer parts of the country.) Since thrushes have the habit of looking for sprouted seeds and earthworms in the planter boxes, keep the containers covered until the grass has become a green carpet. When you grow it outside, you may need to be more patient especially during the spring and autumn until the cereal grass is ready to be harvested after two to four weeks.

The makers of barley grass powder say that it is not possible for the barley grass grown at home to have the same nutrient concentration as that grown outside. At home, the barley grass never reaches the important jointing stage, a point in time when the seed pushes into the blade and can be recognized by a thickening. At this time, the nutrient concentration in the barley grass is the highest: all simple sugars have been converted into complex carbohydrates. For example, the barley for one maker's barley grass preparation is grown in prairie soil rich in minerals. It is sown in the autumn and harvested in the spring, which means it has a slow growth process of almost 200 days behind it. Barley grass and wheat grass from the windowsill taste sweeter, which can be explained by the high portion of simple sugars.

I personally use both methods. The fresh, self-grown cereal grass certainly also has many nutrients and vital substances since Dr. Ann Wigmore would otherwise not have had such sensational success in healing many diseases in her institute. Moreover, I take advantage of the abundance of vital substances in the barley grass powder from the jar and also take barley grass powder tablets that are pressed at low temperatures when I travel, in addition to my own homegrown grass. I invite you to experiment and discover what tastes better and agrees better with you. Perhaps it's better to replace "either-or" thinking with "both-and" thinking!

The Contents of Barley Grass Juice and Their Meaning

Barley Grass Has a Unique Nutrient Profile that is Optimal for Human Beings

Is barley grass the world's richest nutritional source, as Dr. Yoshihide Hagiwara claims? There is much evidence to support this claim. Barley grass is a high-quality food with all of the minerals, enzymes, vitamins (except for vitamin D, which the body creates itself when there is enough sunlight), and all of the vital amino acids, both the essential ones that the body must absorb from the food and the non-essential ones. In comparison to other foods, barley grass contains many times the amount of enzymes, vitamins, and minerals; in comparison to other green plants, it has the highest content of chlorophyll. The only other comparable food in this regard is blue-green algae!

Barley grass juice is not only impressive in terms of the amount of vital substances it contains, but also because of the balanced composition that appears to precisely meet the needs of the human body. Consequently, barley grass appears to be the ideal food supplement of a natural origin for us; it cannot be compared with the effect of vitamin or mineral tablets because the contents occur in a natural composition and have a synergistic effect. Experts believe that there is absolutely no substitute for green food in our diets: If you refuse this "sunlight-energy food," to a great extent you will rob yourself of a very special elixir of life.

Barley Grass Offers an Abundance of Everything

Barley grass juice provides twice as much calcium as milk, twice as much calcium and potassium as wheat grass, about 30 times more of all the B vitamins than milk, as well as the important vitamin B12 and abundant provitamin A (beta carotene), and seven times as much vitamin C as the corresponding amount of oranges, five times as much iron as spinach, and large amounts of the important minerals magnesium, potassium, copper, and zinc. According to Halima Neumann, this nutrient profile cannot be offered by any animal food. Barley grass contains isoflavonoids that have an effect similar to that of certain endogenous estrogens in the body. These are particularly significant for the prevention of osteoporosis since they retain calcium and promote the depositing of calcium in the bones. In addition, isoflavonoids support the regeneration of the skin.

Barley grass contains a high portion of essential fatty acids such as linoleic acid and linolenic acid. These essential fatty acids participate in the production of prostaglandin, hormone-like substances, and accelerate the speed of cell growth, improve the condition of the skin, and support the functioning of the liver. Moreover, they stimulate the activity of the endocrine glands and strengthen the nervous system. The fatty acids contained in barley grass consist of about 50% linolenic acid, 20% palmitic acid, and 9% linoleic acid.

Here is a summary of the amounts of other foods necessary to be the equivalent of the components in three grams—about one teaspoon—of barley grass powder:

Nutrient[34]	Milk (ml)	Lettuce (g)	Tomatoes (g)
Potassium	167.0	128.3	92.7
Calcium	167.0	158.6	1,110.0
Carotene			
(incl. provit. A)	1,300.0	158.6	390.3
Vitamin B2	55.0	138.0	275.0
Vitamin C	492.3	200.0	49.2

As a food supplement taken two to three times a day, Dr. Yoshihide Hagiwara recommends a dosage of one g of barley grass powder for babies, two to six g (approx. one to two teaspoons) for schoolchildren, and double this amount for people with symptoms or a tendency toward hyperacidity (acidosis).

As a food supplement, barley grass is more relevant than ever. Dr. Yoshihide Hagiwara says in "Green Barley Essence" that: the green barley extract can be an antidote for the increasingly deteriorating nutrition of the fast-food culture because it is a very natural fast food and still has a higher content of the five essential nutrients (minerals, vitamins, proteins, chlorophyll, and enzymes) than any other natural food. Dr. Mary Ruth Swope recommends barley grass powder as the sole food supplement since it contains all of the substances required by the body in an optimal composition.

Nutrient Profile of Barley Grass Powder

10 g of barley grass powder contain 2288 mg protein, 1716 mg raw fiber, 53 mg chlorophyll, 4 g carbohydrates, and just 29 calories.

Minerals		Amino Acids		Vitamins[35]	
Calcium	52 mg	Lysine	83 mg	Vitamin A	5005 IU
Manganese	1 mg	Aspartic acid	223 mg	E (tocopherol)	3 mg
Zinc	50 mcg	Proline	94 mg	B2 (riboflavin)	203 mcg
Cobalt	5 mcg	Valine	126 mg	B3 (niacin)	752 mcg
Phosphorus	52 mg	Tyrosine	52 mg	B1 (thiamine)	29 mcg
Selenium	10 mcg	Cystine	23 mg	B6 (pyrodoxine)	129 mcg
Iodine	20 mcg	Purine	6 mg	B12 (cobalamin)	3 mcg
Sulfur	20 mg	Histidine	46 mg	Folic acid	109 mcg
Potassium	320 mcg	Threonine	106 mg	Vitamin K	801 mcg
Sodium	3 mg	Glycine	117 mg	Pantothenic	
Copper	6 mg	Isoleucine	89 mg	acid	240 mcg
(and approx. 80 more		Phenylalanine	11 mg	C (ascorbic	
trace elements with a		Serine	243 mg	acid)	32 mg
total of 369 mg)		Arginine	112 mg	Choline	3 mg
		Glutaminic		Biotin	11 mcg
		acid	243 mg		
		Alanine	137 mg		
		Leucine	163 mg		
		Methionine	43 mg		
		Amidine	29 mg		

Optimally Usable Proteins in Barley Grass

Plant Protein in Barley Grass

The juice from young barley plants is one of the oldest healing remedies known to humanity. Even the Essenes of Jesus' age used the power of barley and wheat grass. It contains all the nutrients that we need to live in a balanced concentration. It should especially be emphasized that barley grass juice and the powder that is made from it has a high protein content, which is 45% of the weight of barley grass powder. As a result, it is the largest individual component of this food. In comparison: whole-wheat flour contains only 10% protein, milk 3%, eggs 12%, and steak 16%.

Barley grass is a complete, high-quality source of protein with about 23% protein in the fresh juice. Ronald L. Seibold states that the protein in cereal grasses is superior to any other plant source of protein. The idea that protein from animals is especially healthy is a prejudice. Quite the opposite is true: The protein in meat, for example, requires a long time for digestion and often leaves protein residue in the intestines, which can become the trigger for allergies and other health disorders.

When digesting protein from an animal source, the body requires an unnecessarily high amount of energy to make its own amino acids. The idea that only steaks create big muscles is an erroneous belief

On the other hand, the body can use up to about 90% of the easily digestible protein molecules from plants. This occurs without—like meat—leaving behind any of the waste products like purines and uric acids that contribute to hyperacidity of the body (acidosis). Acidosis creates an "acidic breeding ground," the over-acidified body environment that promotes the development of many diseases like rheumatism or diabetes, as well as cancer (see "Restoring the Acid-Alkaline Balance with Barley Grass Juice," page 96). The excess consumption of proteins from animal sources by the general public is related to the development of various types of cancer, especially breast cancer and intestinal cancer.

Proteins, which consist of about twenty amino acids, form the supporting structural framework of the body and participate in the composition of the cell walls, connective tissue, muscles, enzymes, and various membranes. The meaning of proteins becomes clear when we remember that enzymes participate in all of the life processes and that some proteins also work as hormones and regulators of the metabolic processes. Protein is part of every living cell; without protein, it would not be possible for the body cells to live.

Ronald L. Seibold believes that the meaning of an appropriate supply of protein in nutrition cannot be overemphasized. As functional components of muscle tissue, antibodies, hormones, enzymes, and cellular membranes, proteins are involved in practically every metabolic reaction of the body including repair and renewal of tissue, energy production, immune function, neural activity, digestion, etc.

All Essential Amino Acids Available in Barley Grass

The body requires all eight of the essential amino acids that are not endogenious (produced by the body itself) in very specific proportions in order to build healthy tissue. Essential amino acids must therefore be given to it through the diet. If just one of the essential amino acids is missing or just present in an inadequate amount in a meal, the organism is not capable of forming the cell-building substances for its tissue from the rest of the amino acids. It is therefore especially important for vegetarians, vegans, raw-foodists, and fruitarians to add complete plant proteins from plants such as barley grass or blue-green algae, either fresh or in powder form at a dosage of ten to twenty grams (one to two teaspoons), to meals since many plant proteins are "incomplete." Grain, for example, contains the lowest value of the essential amino acid lysine, while beans often are lacking in methionine. In contrast to most plant proteins, barley grass contains a high proportion of methionine, as well as lysine.

Barley grass contains abundant quantities of the amino acid tryptophan, from which our brain produces serotonin, a neurotransmitter known to play a critical role in mood. We require a high level of serotonin in order to learn well, experience joy in life, and be cheerful. If the serotonin level is too low, we may suffer from mood fluctuations, depression, feelings of anxiety, difficulties in learning and concentrating, and sleep disorders. In the evening, the body transforms the serotonin in the body into melatonin and we can fall asleep more easily. Furthermore, serotonin supports the contraction of smooth muscle cells.

However, we shouldn't eat any solid foods after 6 p.m. because "the intestines go to sleep with the chickens." Instead, it's best to limit ourselves to fluid foods like freshly squeezed fruit juices and barley grass juice or blue-green algae drinks. Simply mix one heaping teaspoon of barley grass and/or blue-green algae into a glass of non-carbonated water. You can find additional ideas for mixed barley grass drinks in the recipe section of this book.

Good for the Brain and the Mood!

Barley grass contains substantial amounts of other important amino acids as well. One hundred grams of barley grass juice powder contains approximately 240 mg of glutamic acid, an amino acid important for neural transmission, and 110 mg of phenylalanine. The latter amino acid promotes vitality and mental agility, as well as reducing depression, pain, and feelings of hunger.

Barley grass juice contains all of the essential and non-essential amino acids in a balanced composition and in a stable state. The essential amino acids isoleucine, leucine, lysine, methionine, phenylalanine, threonine, trypthophan, and valine are contained in barley grass juice, as well as the amino acids alanine, arginine, aspartic acid, glutamic acid, glycine, histidine, proline, serine, tyrosine, and cystine. From arginine, the body produces the human growth hormone (HGH), which is responsible for the formation of cartilage, among other things. Increased production of arginine can help ease intervertebral disk problems and related backache. There is also an ample supply of arginine in papayas.[36]

Enzymes are a key to longevity.
(Dr. Mary Ruth Swope in "Green Leaves of Barley")

Barley grass is an excellent source of all essential amino acids and many other others in an optimally usable form. As a result, it is absolutely necessary as a regular component of the diet for athletes, sick persons, brainworkers and creative individuals, pregnant women, children, vegans, and people with a high level of stress since all of these groups have an increased need for high-quality protein.

Dr. Mary Ruth Swope does not make a secret of her enthusiasm about the nutrient profile of green barley grass. She believes that the nutritional advantages of barley make it a super-aristocrat in the family of grains. Time and again, she emphasizes that cell health is true prosperity.[37] Dr. Yoshihide Hagiwara recommends preferring green barley grass as a source of protein over milk products and meat because it is more easily available to the body and does not burden it with fat and cholesterol.

Barley Grass:
a "Treasure Chest" Full of Enzymes

Enzymes, Heat-Sensitive "Sparks" of Life

Enzymes are the "sparks" of life. Without enzymes, there would be no life and no organism could survive! Digestion, as well as respiration, cell division, as well as thought processes and the healing of wounds are all dependent upon the activity of the enzymes. The enzymes within the organism have the effect of biological catalysts that activate and control the chemical reactions. They consist of protein and are true marvels that do not consume themselves during their activities.

In order to become active, enzymes require a specific pH environment and certain vitamins, minerals, and trace elements as coenzymes and cofactors, as participants. These vital substances (above all, the B vitamins) help the enzymes in their work and are used up in the process, so they must be supplied to the body in adequate amounts. Barley grass not only contains a great many enzymes, but also the related coenzymes that we normally no longer receive in adequate amounts with the customary diet.

More than 700 enzymes in the human body have now been identified and characterized to a large degree in terms of structure and function but scientists hypothesize that there are thousands of enzymes remaining to be identified. Even in one single liver cell, more than one-thousand enzyme systems are active. For more information, including the discovery of what role enzymes play in our health, see my book *Healing Power of Papaya*.

Enzymes are sensitive to heat. Many "die" even at temperatures above 42 degrees C. When we eat raw, unprocessed foods, they provide the enzymes that play similar roles to the body's own enzymes, including digestive enzymes. Tropical fruits such as papayas and pineapples are especially rich in enzymes and they contain an abundance of the enzymes papain or bromelain. In addition to fresh fruit, enzyme tablets made from fruit can also supply these enzymes. These are commercially available in a high-dosage, enzyme-active quality of a natural origin.

Cooked, fried, or baked food no longer contains any enzymes. Dr. Mary Ruth Swope points out that about 65% of the food offered in American supermarkets has been heated and is therefore worthless in terms of enzymes. Since the pancreas must make more digestive enzymes available for denatured food, it becomes prematurely exhausted. This results in problems with the pancreas, premature aging, and weakening of the immune system.[38]

We can imagine enzymes as protein-bearers, charged with vital energy; but like the batteries of a flashlight, this energy can be exhausted and we must learn to conserve and recharge it. Cooked foods exhaust the glands that produce enzymes, but raw plant foods stimulate them.

A Low Level of Enzymes Allow
Health Disorders to Develop

Some physicians, like the German Dr. Hans Nieper at the Silbersee Clinic in Hanover, use enzymes, in addition to a strict vegetarian diet, to fight degenerative disorders like cancer, heart disease, diabetes, and arteriosclerosis. Many researchers now call enzymes the "key to a long life." Remember: Without enzymes, there is no digestion and no assimilation; without complete digestion and assimilation, there is no radiant health; and without enzymes, there is no resistance to deadly diseases.

Barley Grass, One of the Best Sources of Enzymes

Barley grass juice is an excellent source of enzymes, probably one of the best there is. Dr. Mary Ruth Swope writes that the green leaves of the young barley plants are an excellent source of hundreds of 'living' enzymes," ("Green Leaves of Barley") in contrast to vitamin or mineral tablets from the chemistry laboratory. More than 80 enzymes have now been identified in barley grass, but it probably contains hundreds of them. Among the enzymes found in barley green, cytochrome oxidase, superoxide dimutase (SOD), peroxidase, and catalase should be mentioned in particular. These enzymes are extremely important in order to avoid the premature aging of cells and dissolve cancer-causing substances.

This book contains a separate chapter on "SOD—A Wonder Remedy?" (See page 94 ff.) Peroxidase is also capable of stimulating the regeneration of damaged DNA in the nucleus of the cell and breaks down hydrogen peroxide. Catalase is capable of splitting cell-damaging hydrogen peroxide (H_2O_2) into water and oxygen as a by-product of the respiratory process, making it harmless as a result. This is why catalase is successfully used as an immune-strengthening treatment for cancer patients. Cytochrome oxidase catalyzes the oxygen reduction and transhydrogenase exercises an important function in the muscle tissue of the heart. All of the enzymes mentioned here are "responsible" for the removal of fat; when we don't consume enough of them, weight problems can develop. Furthermore, they dissolve the toxic substances within the body that lead to health disorders.

Dr. Yoshihide Hagiwara describes barley grass as a "treasure chest full of enzymes."[39]

Dr. Mary Ruth Swope writes: "It is wonderful that nature makes a food available to us, namely barley grass, that through enzymes and coenzymes (in addition to amino acids, minerals, chlorophyll, etc.) has the power to provide our cells with the fundamental weapons required for health, as well as for fighting disease." ("Green Leaves of Barley".) Even if you just add several teaspoons of dried barley grass juice to your diet every day, you would certainly improve your quality of life. Barley grass is the food with enzyme power!

Barley Grass,
a Cornucopia of Vital Vitamins

Barley Grass, a Healthy Alternative to Pills

The meaning of vitamins as guardians for our health is generally known. They play an important role in the metabolism by participating in significant chemical reactions as coenzymes. In addition, vitamins strengthen our immune system; certain vitamins, like vitamin C, vitamin E, and provitamin A act as "antioxidants" against the cell-destroying effect of the free radicals, aggressive oxygen compounds and thereby slow down the aging process.

Even individuals who have a healthy diet with large amounts of fruit and vegetables should remember that the vitamin content of our foods is constantly decreasing because of the cultivation methods of industrial agriculture, the exhaustion of the soil, and lengthy transportation routes, and the overly long storage that does not preserve the vitamins, as well as the thoughtless "overcooking" at home and elsewhere. "You Must Be Kidding: An Apple a Day!" was the heading of an article in the German magazine *Bio* (about natural living) in August of 1998 with the bad news that the vitamin C content of apples had been reduced by 80% in the last ten years. "The situation is not much better for other types of fruits and vegetables." Accordingly, the content of beta carotene in fennel also shrunk by 80% during this time period; the calcium content of broccoli was reduced to one-third, and carrots now contain just one-fourth as much magnesium as they did ten years ago because of increasing stress and environmental toxins.[40]

However, our need for vitamins has increased during this time. Deficiencies of vital substances are pre-programmed in this situation. In order to prevent diseases and symptoms of premature aging, it is therefore necessary to additionally supply the body with large doses of organic and naturally occurring food supplements that are not isolated. A food supplement like barley grass, which gives us all the vitamins we need together with other vital substances like minerals and enzymes in a high concentration and natural balance, can be highly recommended.

The Body Only Absorbs
Natural Vitamins

In recent years, many health enthusiasts have become "crazy" about vitamin pills. But vitamins, especially those that have been isolated and chemically produced, can create an imbalance in the sensitive equilibrium of the body. Dr. Yoshihide Hagiwara believes that vitamins must be natural and not synthetic in order to promote health. Many physicians warn against taking isolated and synthetically manufactured vitamins because they are poorly absorbed by the body or may even have a toxic effect when higher dosages are taken.[41] Dr. Ann Wigmore criticizes taking isolated vitamins because "too much" can also confuse the overall nutrient balance within the body. She believes that the antioxidants that we find in food additives can also be found in wheat grass and other natural foods but here they are more efficient than the chemically extracted substances.[42]

Synthetically produced vitamins are viewed as foreign substances by the body, which sends them to the liver for detoxification; the residue is then either eliminated through the kidneys or stored in the fat cells as toxins. Americans are famous for their high consumption of vitamin pills; a colorful arsenal of mostly synthetically produced pills is already on their breakfast table. Dr. Richard Gold, from Pacific College of Oriental Medicine in San Diego, California says that Americans take mega-doses of vitamins and that they have the reputation of having the 'most expensive' urine in the world. Although the American population has the highest per capita spending for health care in the world, they are only number 27 on the list of countries with the highest life expectancy.

Natural foods like barley grass contain hundreds of components that combine synergistically and support each other as they do their work in our digestive system and bloodstream. Consequently, calcium and pyridoxine are necessary for the absorption of vitamin B12, which is important for the activation of folic acid; furthermore, iron is required to transform beta carotene into vitamin A. All of the substances mentioned here, and others necessary for an optimum metabolism, are contained in barley grass. Barley grass powder has been used in the USA and Japan for more than sixty years as a natural vitamin and mineral food supplement with only positive results, even when taken for decades and at a high dosage.

All Vitamins in a Balanced Relationship

The vitamin content of barley grass juice is astonishing. With the exception of vitamin D, which is produced by the body itself in the skin with the help of sunlight, it contains all of the vitamins; these are in a concentrated and balanced form, just as the body requires them. Barley green (dried barley grass juice) contains all the vitamins of the B group and about 30 times as many B vitamins as milk, as well as the important nerve vitamin B12, six times more provitamin C than apples (330 mg per 100 g), seven times as much provitamin A as spinach (51,500 mg per 100 g), about nine times as much folic acid as spinach (630 mg per 100 g), and many more B vitamins than bananas (1.3 mg B1, 2.7 mg B2, 0.04 mg B4).

Provitamin A, which is converted into vitamin A within the body and also has the function of protecting cells in the form of beta carotene, is important for the optimum functioning of the eyes, the skin, and the mucous membranes. It also protects against sunburn and the harmful effect of carcinogenic (cancer-causing) substances, as well as certain types of cancer such as skin cancer, lung cancer, and ovarian cancer. In addition, it protects us against infections by stimulating the production of antibodies such as T and B lymphocytes. It is also important for body growth and normal bone development. Vitamin A is required for the synthesis of DNA and RNA, as well as for the production of adrenalin. Moreover, it is important for the fertility of women and men. In contrast to vitamin A, which can become toxic in the body at excessive dosages, provitamin A cannot be overdosed. The body only converts as much provitamin A into vitamin A as it needs at the moment. Barley grass can be considered a concentrated food source for beta carotene.

Vitamin K was discovered in 1935 and is normally produced by the body itself when the intestinal flora in the large intestine is healthy. But who has healthy intestinal flora in this day and age? This vitamin is required for the synthesis of important proteins, which are involved in the metabolism of the bones, among other processes, including the ability of the blood to clot. During the 1930s and 1940s, some patients in the USA were successfully given barley grass powder before operations to ensure an adequate supply of vitamin K.[44] This vitamin is also important for women with menstrual problems because it prevents cramps and stops excessive bleeding. Stress uses up vitamin K. Today, more than half of all senior citizens are deficient in vitamin K. Synthetically produced vitamin K is toxic at higher dosages. Cereal grasses like barley grass are the best source of vitamin K.

Barley grass is also an excellent source of natural vitamin C. Among other things, **vitamin C** is important for a strong immune system, the healing of wounds, and the formation of scar tissues. Together with other antioxidants like vitamin E, beta carotene, and selenium, it functions as a catcher of free radicals (oxygen compounds that have a cell-destroying effect). Free radicals participate in the development of degenerative diseases like cancer and premature aging processes. Vitamin C also improves the absorption of iron and calcium. Stress is a vitamin-C thief. Especially smokers, older people, pregnant women, nursing mothers, women who take contraceptive pills, and those who have stressful lives should take advantage of an additional natural source of vitamin C like barley grass.

Folic acid, which is abundantly present in barley grass, has a significant role in the formation, maturation, and regeneration of red blood cells. It also participates in the synthesis of proteins like hemoglobin and is important for our nervous system. Moreover, folic acid is necessary for the synthesis of DNA and RNA. The best sources for folic acid are dark-green leafy vegetables such as barley grass. Since we generally eat too little of this food in general, a deficiency in folic acid is widespread. About 60% of all women have an inadequate supply of this substance. Especially during pregnancy, a dangerous folic-acid deficiency can occur. This may lead to deformities of the newborn or miscarriages. Dr. Yoshihide Hagiwara recommends that pregnant women take at least two teaspoons of barley grass powder dissolved in water as a preventive measure. Symptoms of folic-acid deficiency can be anemia, digestive disorders, torn corners of the mouth, and irritability.

Vitamin B12 is required by the body in order to convert folic acid from the inactive to an active form. In addition, this vitamin is important for healthy nerve tissue and the formation of blood cells. It also participates in the fat and protein metabolism. A vitamin-B12 deficiency can manifest itself through a lack of energy. Since vegetarians and vegans do not have any animal sources of vitamin B12, such as meat and milk products, it is recommended that they use a plant source of vitamin B12 as a food supplement, namely barley grass or wheat grass.

Important for vegetarians and vegans: Barley grass is one of the few plant sources of vitamin B12!

Vitamin B6 (pyridoxine) is important for the synthesis of numerous proteins. It acts like a coenzyme in the body during the processing of carbohydrates and fats. Furthermore, pyridoxine is important for the formation of neurotransmitters, which send impulses through the brain and nervous system. It is also responsible for the formation of antibodies. Pyridoxine cannot be stored by the body. However, on the average, Americans have less than the seventy percent of the recommended amounts of vitamin B6 in their diets. A deficiency of pyridoxine can be expressed in anemia, irritability, sleep disorders, and the formation of kidney stones. Barley grass is one of the best sources of pyridoxine. Together with its additional components of vitamin C, vitamin B12, folic acid, and iron, it supports the maintenance of a healthy immune system and a healthy hemoglobin level.

A type of vitamin E, **alpha-tocopherol succinate**, was discovered in barley grass in 1994. This substance promotes the release of prolactin, as well as a growth hormone, through the cells of the pituitary gland. Prolactic, an ingredient of breast milk, has a very calming, mood-brightening effect and supports emotional equilibrium. According to recent research, violent criminals have an unusually low level of prolactin. Studies have shown that prolactin reduces aggressiveness and strengthens the immune system through the increased production of white blood cells. In addition, prolactin helps delay aging processes and maintain healthy tissues, healthy brain cells, and healthy bones even during the senior years. Furthermore, alpha-tocopherol reduces the risk of breast cancer and cancer of the colon. It prevents the growth of cancer cells ten times as effectively as normal vitamin E, which is well-known for its cancer-preventing effect.

Minerals, the "Core of Life"

Our Soil's Mineral Deficiency Threatens Our Health

As I write this chapter, I am living on the Canary Island of La Palma. Just twenty years ago, a volcano was spitting fire and it may erupt again at any time. Magma—with its abundance of minerals like iron, magnesium, potassium, and zinc—poured over the island and into the ocean. Once it hardened, it created the most fertile soil that we can imagine. If we just let the severed crown of a pineapple fall on the ground, a new pineapple plant will grow from it in a matter of days. The carrots that grow in a girlfriend's garden here taste so sweet and intensive—even organic carrots from my own garden don't taste this good in Germany.

Increasingly more of the minerals that are important for our health are being washed into the rivers and oceans. Could it be that the Japanese have the longest life expectancy among the industrial nations because they bring these minerals back to their plates through the vegetables of the sea-algae?

In earlier ages, when there were volcanic eruptions all over the entire planet, the mineral-enriched earth was washed into the oceans by the rainfall. The first primitive life arose in such a mineral-saturated ocean. Consequently, Dr. Yoshihide Hagiwara calls the minerals as the core of physical life.[45] The plants that cover the earth today still contain, just like the primal oceans of that period, more potassium than salt. The ion equilibrium has apparently hardly changed since then. Our blood has about the same salt and mineral content as the seas.

Dr. Mary Ruth Swope says: "If you are constantly tired because of a potassium-deficiency, try green barley grass juice and observe whether or not this makes a difference. I have already had a "good" diet for years, but barley grass extract still gives me more energy—and I believe that it will also help you." ("Green Leaves of Barley")

Minerals are just as important for our health as vitamins. Many vitamins can only fulfill their tasks with the help of minerals. Chinese medicines therefore contain many minerals with the goal of restoring the equilibrium of minerals in our cells and stimulating the life processes. Dr. Mary Ruth Swope writes that enzymes, catalysts that make the metabolism possible, only work when the right minerals are released into our cellular fluid as ions. As a result, Dr. Mary Ruth Swope called minerals "the enzymes for the enzymes." Minerals play an important role in metabolism and are a component of every cell. They must constantly be replaced because they are continually eliminated through the urine, sweat, and stools.[47]

The only source from which we can supply ourselves with the necessary *organic* minerals and trace elements is our food, and the most important source of minerals are fruits and vegetables. According to Dr. Yoshihide Hagiwara, when we neglect to eat foods with the right mineral content, the body cannot blossom.

Minerals Are Important for Our Acid-Alkaline Balance

Minerals are very important for the regulation of the acid-alkaline balance (also see the chapter in this book on "Restoring the Acid-Alkaline Balance with Barley Grass Juice" on page 96 ff.). They promote the ability of the muscles to contract and participate in the excitability of the nervous system: more **potassium** has a stimulating effect on the vagus nerve, and an increase in calcium stimulates the sympathetic nervous system. Both regulate the effect of hormones; potassium weakens the effect of adrenaline. Potassium, abundantly present in barley grass, supports healthy functioning of the intestines by stimulating peristalsis (intestinal movement) in a natural way, as well as contributing to the composition and maintenance of the sphincter muscles.

Our food generally contains much more sodium than potassium. As a result, our acid-alkaline balance is shifted to the acidic side and we are constantly "in the red" because our "account" is overdrawn and in the "acidic minus" area.[46] The balance of potassium and sodium is indispensable for maintaining the osmotic equilibrium, the regulation of the water balance in every cell. Sufficient potassium is also necessary for a calm heartbeat; it reduces the blood pressure and therefore also the risk of a heart attack or stroke. Continuing diarrhea and extended use of laxatives, as well as eating disorders such as bulimia, lead to a potassium deficiency. Many women over the age of 60 are dependent on laxatives, which cause the intestinal muscles to slacken in the long run and dangerously rob the body of its minerals.

The Minerals in Barley Grass Strengthen Our Immune System and Keep Us Healthy

Zinc, which is amply present in barley grass, is important for our immune system and the action of about 200 enzymes. Like the trace element **manganese** (which is also found in barley grass), it is also important for insulin storage, the healing of wounds, and the coordination of the nerves, the brain, and muscle activity. In addition, manganese is required for the formation of cartilage tissue and can prevent the feared degeneration of the intervertebral disks. Manganese is also an important factor in the metabolism of protein, fat, and sugar. Zinc, like manganese, normalizes the blood-sugar level and is essential for the functioning of muscles and nerve cells. A manganese deficiency has been discovered in the blood of women who suffer from osteoporosis. Zinc is employed against skin diseases, and even the ancient Egyptians also used it against emotional disorders.[47]

The heart and muscles profit in particular from **magnesium**, which is amply present in barley grass. It is important for strengthening the heart, as well as being a vital nerve and muscle relaxant. Heart-attack patients who receive magnesium therapy have much better chances of survival. In addition, it is employed in accompanying cancer therapy and also plays a role in preventing cancer. Even the soil used for organic cultivation is often exhausted and only has a minimum of magnesium.

Among other symptoms, people who suffer from a lack of magnesium are quick to react in an irritated manner and are susceptible to stress. Magnesium protects not only the heart, but also keeps the bones healthy by ensuring that the calcium reaches the bones. The body needs magnesium to form the enzymes required for the development of stable bone-mineral crystals. Without the vitamins B1 and B6, which are also present in barley grass, the body cannot properly absorb and use magnesium.

The important trace element **copper** can also be found in barley grass. Like zinc, copper is an essential component of many of our body's enzymes and therefore indispensable for numerous vital processes in the organism. This trace element is also a decisive factor in protecting us against anemia and arteriosclerosis. Without copper, iron cannot be stored in the blood. Copper plays an important role in the immune system by promoting the formation of antibodies and the so-called killer T cells. Furthermore, copper is the main element for the pigmentation of skin and hair. It protects us against graying prematurely and sallow, pale skin. Taking too much zinc will cause the level of copper in the blood to decrease, and vice versa. Both of these substances exist in a balanced relationship in barley grass.

Barley grass juice contains more **iron** than spinach. Iron is important for the formation of blood. However, iron cannot form hemoglobin (the red blood pigment) without adequate copper. Like all dark-green plant juices, barley grass contains copper and iron in an ideal relationship in order to ensure the best-possible absorption.

In barley grass, there are also abundant amounts of calcium that the body can optimally utilize. This substance supports the relaxation of the heart muscle and keeps the bones hard and stable. Our bones contain about one kilo (2.2 pounds) of calcium and the body also eliminates calcium every day; as a result, we must take in about one gram of calcium through our food on a daily basis. Under the keyword "Osteoporosis" in the A - Z section of this book, there is an explanation of why the calcium contained in plants like barley grass is much more valuable for the body than the calcium found in milk products. Ronald L. Seibold says that osteoporosis is practically unknown in many of the world's countries where milk products are rarely eaten.[48] In barley grass, the calcium is bound to proteins and therefore can be absorbed much more easily by the body than through calcium tablets, for example. The absorption of calcium in the body requires estrogen. Estrogen-like substances, isoflavonoids, are present in barley grass.

Many members of the medical profession consider the lack of selenium in our soil and in the human blood serum to be responsible for the increase in cancer cases. **Selenium** is an antioxidant and protects us against free radicals and environmental toxins like cadmium, lead, and nitrite. This mineral even reduces the toxicity of mercury in the body. Individuals with a high level of selenium are better protected against invaders like viruses and bacteria. Patients who are negatively effected by the environment, people suffering from rheumatism, and cancer patients have a dramatically lowered level of selenium. Increasingly more members of the medical profession are therefore demanding that the selenium level be constantly monitored in people who are chronically ill; in cases of deficiency, the level should then be raised with the help of food supplements.

Dr. Yoshihide Hagiwara believes that the imbalance of minerals in the cells causes numerous health disorders. With its unique spectrum of vital substances, barley grass is the ideal, balanced, and natural food supplement for eliminating mineral deficiencies.

A Unique Antioxidant in Barley Grass

Oxygen Can Also Destroy

There are "good" and "bad" types of oxygen. The latter types are quick to react and can cause various diseases, including cancer, diabetes, arteriosclerosis, inflammations, immune weakness, and premature aging. Many of these "bad" types of oxygen are man-made and can be found in cigarette smoke, automobile exhaust, pesticides, industrial plants, and the smoke created by forest fires (this information comes from a lecture by Professor Shibamoto in Germany on Oct. 10, 1998).

Ultraviolet (UV) light also produces "bad" oxygen that is harmful to health. It is therefore important to supply our bodies with oxidants such as natural vitamin E, vitamin C, and selenium in order to get rid of the "bad" oxygen and also protect our cells against oxidative destruction.

In addition to the many anti-oxidative enzymes such as SOD, catalyse, and peroxidase, barley grass contains an isoflavonoid that was just discovered in 1992 with the name of 2"-O-glycosylisovitexin. Its abbreviation is 2"-O-GIV. Barley grass juice contains about 0.5% to 0.7% 2"-O-GIV. This is a unique, extremely effective antioxidant that hasn't been found to date in any other food. It prevents the oxidation of lipids in our cells, thereby hindering premature aging and symptoms of degeneration.[49]

Two studies from the year 1992 carried out (s. Bibliography on pg. 145-147) by Dr. Yoshihide Hagiwara together with T. Osawa, K. Kitta, and Professor Shibamoto isolated and identified GIV and discovered that it has an antioxidant effect. Antioxidants neutralize

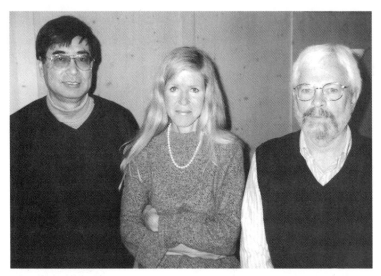

This photo was taken after a lecture by Professor Shibamoto in Munich; Germany, in October 1998. From left to right in the picture: Professor Shibamoto, Barbara Simonsohn, and Dr. Bob Terry, Ph.D., nutrition advisor and manager of Relationship Marketing of "Green Foods Corporation", Oxnard, CA, USA.

free radicals that lead to the oxidation of lipids (fats). In this process, malonaldehyde (MA) is formed. The less MA, the more effectively the antioxidant prevents the formation of lipid peroxides in our cells. Lipid peroxides are very reactive oxygen compounds (the scientific studies are listed in the Bibliography on pages 147-148).

The antioxidant 2"-O-GIV may owe part of its effectiveness to being both water- and fat-soluble. Cellular membranes are composed of an outer layer that is receptive to water-soluble soluble substances and an inner layer that is receptive to fat-soluble substances. Since most antioxidants are either water-soluble (e.g. vitamin C) or fat-soluble (e.g. beta-carotene or vitamin E) but not both, they only have access to either the outer or inner portions of the cellular membrane. Hypothetically, 2"-O-GIV may be able to traverse both the outer and inner layers of the cellular membrane, thereby offering greater antioxidant protection than antioxidants with more limited solubility.

Glycolsylsovitexin Is More Effective
than Vitamin E

In 1993, Tadashi Nishiyama (s. Bibliography on page 148) studied the effect of 2"-O-GIV and vitamin E (alpha-tocopherol) on the development of MA formation. This study came to the conclusion that vitamin E is destroyed under UV radiation, but not 2"-O-GIV. This substance is 500 times as effective as a cell-protecting remedy than the potent antioxidant vitamin E and even exceeds the cell-protecting effect of lecithin and cod-liveroil. In view of the increasing UV radiation because of the ozone hole, and with the subsequent danger of developing skin cancer, this study has a special significance.

A study published in 1994 in the magazine *Food Phytochemicals for Cancer Prevention II* came to the conclusion that 2"-O-GIV had a substantially higher antioxidant effect than vitamin E, beta carotene, and a 60% methanol solution against dangerous, cancer-causing barbiturates.

The substance 2"-O-GIV is soluble in water and alcohol, and stable even at high temperatures up to 100 degrees C. It develops its effect in a broad pH spectrum of pH 3 to pH 9. As protection against oxidation of the blood plasma, 2"-O-GIV is more effective than vitamin E and almost as effective as Probucol, a medication that lowers blood pressure and has side-effects. Professor Shibamoto considers 2"-O-GIV to be the ideal preventive "medicine" as prophylaxis against arteriosclerosis since he believes that the oxidation of LDL (which is prevented by this antioxidant) is responsible for this disease. He believes that 2"-O-GIV potentially offers greater potential against arteriosclerosis than the synthetic drug, Probucol.

We are constantly, 24 hours a day, subject to the effects of "bad" oxygen from our surrounding world. Statistics show the drastic increase of diseases such as skin cancer, asthma, candida, arthritis, and so forth. Even if we eat a healthy diet, our body must deal with environmental toxins like automobile exhaust, air pollution, cigarette smoke, household chemicals, and toxins in new clothing. In order to have the type of protection that we need, it is therefore very important to continually take a natural supplement like barley grass powder with its powerful antioxidants on a regular basis. The newly discovered barley grass antioxidant 2"-O-GIV appears to play an outstanding role as a cell-protecting remedy in the prevention of premature aging processes and chronic diseases.

THE HEALING EFFECT
OF BARLEY GRASS

Chlorophyll—A Healing Remedy in Ancient Times

For centuries, the green parts of plants have been used to promote the healing of wounds. Even in ancient times, the greenest plants were preferentially used for healing purposes. During the Twentieth Century, scientists discovered that chlorophyll is an effective deodorant, a competent detoxifier, and a wound-healer.[50] Experts consider chlorophyll to be the most effective method for stimulating the formation of new cells and the repair of tissue. They have shown that the healing of wounds takes place in a substantially shorter time period with chlorophyll therapy than with penicillin, vitamin D, sulphanilamide, or no treatment at all.

Today, chlorophyll tablets are given on a routine basis to elderly patients with digestive problems and incontinence in homes for the aged, by healing practitioners, and in hospitals to reduce odors. Many skin creams and ointments for better wound-healing are now available containing chlorophyll, as well as toothpaste and chewing gum,

As already explained in the chapter on "Chlorophyll, the Blood of Plants," on page 15 ff. chlorophyll is converted to hemoglobin by animal and human bodies. It is therefore quite understandable that this green plant pigment is injected intravenously as a blood-builder to humans and animals for increasing the amount of hemoglobin. In comparison to the chemically produced chlorophyll, the natural form is always more effective and free of side-effects. According to Viktoras Kulvinskas, in cases where this chemical therapy fails or is only temporarily successful, the anemia disappears when the patient receives an organic diet and is provided with chlorophyll in a natural form, as grass juice.[51] Green grass juices are therefore especially recommended as blood-builders for anemic individuals, women during pregnancy, and vegetarians.

Chlorophyll Is Safe to Use

In addition to anemia, chlorophyll has a balancing and healing effect on other ailments. Viktoras Kulvinskas lists the following disorders, for which the healing power of chlorophyll has been demonstrated: [52]

- Lack of protein
- Sinusitis
- Arteriosclerosis
- Stomach ulcer
- Osteomylitis (bacterial infection of the bones)
- Pyorrhea (discharge of pus)
- Peritonitis
- Depression

The discovery of chlorophyll as a healing remedy is not new: as early as 1940, the Journal of Surgery printed a report on more than 12000 cases of illness in which chlorophyll had been successfully used for quickly healing. Even in high doses, chlorophyll is absolutely non-toxic for both animals and human beings. This applies whether it is injected intravenously or intramuscularly or taken orally.

Impressing Healing Success with Barley Grass Powder

In his book, Dr. Yoshihide Hagiwara writes that he did not even consider barley grass to be a medicine or drug for the treatment of specific disorders at the beginning of his research: During a time period of about twenty years, while he introduced Green Barley Essence, "Green Magma" to the Japanese public, he was astonished at its power to improve hundreds of complaints and health problems that had previously not responded to the conventional treatment. Barley grass juice contains 66 times as much chlorophyll as spinach and is therefore one of the best natural sources of chlorophyll. Dr. Yoshihide Hagiwara lists impressive cases of healing success by name, including the following:

- A seventeen-year-old girl who has suffered from asthma and frequent eczemas since childhood. After taking the green barley essence (Green Magma) for one month, the eczema disappeared and the asthma attacks became much less frequent and occurred in a weakened form. After taking the barley grass extract for six months, she hardly had any more asthma attacks and her skin became increasingly smooth and attractive.

- A sixty-year-old woman who had suffered from obesity and high blood pressure not only lost weight: her shoulders, which had been stiff, now became flexible and free of pain.
- A forty-four year-old woman had bad skin and a sallow color to her face. After taking the barley grass juice, her skin became more lively, with a pink color and good circulation. She was very proud that her husband said she looked much younger.
- A fifty-three year-old man was frequently tired, apathetic, and exhausted. What really bothered him: his sexual desire had also fallen asleep. His wife therefore recommended that he take green barley essence. After taking it for six months, he regained his vitality, his abdominal fat melted away, and his sex life became completely normal once again.
- A nineteen-year-old woman suffered from continual constipation and, most likely related symptoms, unrest, irritability, and impatience. Her digestion returned to normal and she also became more mentally stable and capable of making decisions: Now she says that her whole life has changed.
- A man of sixty suffered from a stomach ulcer. After taking Green Magma for just one month, his appetite awakened, he gained nine pounds, and the stomach ulcer healed. Furthermore, his morning nausea disappeared. With Green Barley Essence, he felt he was able to heal the disease from the inside out.
- A fifty-five year-old woman, who had been diagnosed as diabetic, cured her disease solely with natural foods and green barley grass. She believes it is best to heal diabetes through a carefully controlled diet and natural, health-promoting food that improve the constitution.
- A thirty-five year-old woman, who had suffered from high blood pressure since the birth of her third baby, had to stay in bed for three months after the birth because she had intense headaches and a swollen left hand. Her headaches disappeared completely within one month and her blood pressure decreased from 230/130 to 160/100 with Green Magma. In addition, her occasional nose-

bleeds disappeared. Although she had feared that her life would end in her early thirties, it was given to her once again.

Dr. Yoshihide Hagiwara also reports about a fifty-year-old man who could again move his shoulder; a man in his fifties who conquered his heart disease and normalized his blood pressure; a student who overcame his chronically inflamed skin; a forty-year-old man who cured his cirrhosis of the liver after two months with five glasses of barley grass juice every day; and a woman in her late fifties who healed her stomach cancer in the beginning stage and her constipation: She felt even healthier than before her illness, all because of the chlorophyll-containing barley grass juice.

Barley Grass Regenerates the Natural Flow of Energy

On the basis of these experiences, Dr. Yoshihide Hagiwara concludes that the human body itself should be considered the universal remedy. While studying Traditional Chinese Medicine, he had already recognized that its fundamental method is putting the disturbed functions of the human back into their normal state. Just like the therapy with green juices, Chinese herbal medicine is also an appropriate approach for reinstating the natural energy flow in the body instead of focusing on a specific group of symptoms.

This also explains the initially surprising fact that barley grass juice helps against such a wide range of complaints as: skin problems, hair loss, dermatitis, overweight, constipation, hyperacidity, bad breath, inflammations, potency problems, loss of libido, circulatory insufficiency, asthma, irritability, allergies, problems related to the teeth, near-sightedness, high blood pressure, arteriosclerosis, pancreatitis, anemia, leukemia, alcohol problems, flu and colds, inner and outer inflammations, rheumatism and arthritis, Alzheimer's disease, backaches, edemas, osteoporosis, sleep disorders, burns, migraines, multiple sclerosis (MS), depression, menopausal complaints, menstrual problems, stomach ulcers, leg cramps, Parkinson's disease, warts, anacidity (lack of hydrochloric acid), cancer, neurosis, and symptoms of premature aging.[53]

Unfortunately, there isn't space here to discuss more health disorders. More information on this topic can be found in the chapter

"Barley Grass from A to Z" (page 129 ff.). More information about chlorophyll as a cancer-preventing and cancer-healing remedy can be found in the chapter "Barley Grass Against Cancer" on page 108 ff.

Cereal Grass Juices Brake the Growth of Bacteria and Neutralize Toxins

Wheat grass juice and barley grass juice are both rich in chlorophyll, which can be taken orally without any risk. They can also used for enemas in the case of hemorrhoids, for example, or to promote healthy physiological intestinal flora. The antibacterial effect of chlorophyll can apparently be traced to not only the effect that it has on bacteria per se, but also to the creation of an environment that is unfavorable for unhealthy bacteria. Dr. Yoshihide Hagiwara states that he healed his skin infection, which developed because of burning himself with boiling water, solely by brushing barley grass juice onto it.

We all have the opportunity of improving our health by drinking cereal grass juices. I have had very good experiences with both barley grass and wheat grass, fresh and in powder form to be mixed with water. However, if there is a possibility of a candida fungal infestation, only use non-sweet barley grass juice since all sweet foods "feed" the fungus. At the same time, the diet should be changed to include as many fresh (low-sugar) fruits and vegetables as possible.

Human beings die from approximately 250 different diseases while the grass-eating animals like the cow, horse, elephant are only susceptible to five to ten diseases. These animals mainly live from raw, natural foods that Mother Nature provides them and not from ready-made meals, packaged products, and junk food from the factory.

Superoxide Dismutase:
A "Wonder Remedy"?

Barley Grass, One of the Few Sources of SOD

Barley grass provides one of the richest plant sources for the rare enzyme superoxide dismutase (SOD). This enzyme has been found in a wide range of animals, from earthworms to humans, and its function is to neutralize the superoxide ion produced during energy metabolism, thereby preventing the formation of hydrogen peroxide, a source of free radicals. SOD is so critical to the organism's survival that a deficiency of it will lead to an early death, whereas several different types of animals including earthworms, fruit flies, and rats have had their life span dramatically increased by increasing the amount of SOD that their cells produce. It was first discovered and isolated in the blood of a cow in 1969 by professor I. Freedvich at Duke University and J.M. McCord at the University of Southern Alabama. Today, it is presumed that SOD slows down the aging process of the body cells, even in the brain, destroying free radicals as a potent antioxidant. It may be a key to longevity.

Health-conscious people in the USA have made SOD a popular dietary supplement, but most of the SOD available on the American market comes from calf's liver. This practice is questionable in terms of health because many calves in the USA have steroids injected into them in order to quickly build up their muscle mass. A completely safe source of plant SOD is available to us in barley grass juice. Barley grass is the most potent natural source of superoxide dismutase.

How does the enzyme superoxide dismutase act in the human body? Up to now, three different types of SOD have been discovered: a SOD enzyme that contains one copper and one zinc atom; one that contains manganese; and one that contains iron. Erythrocytes (red blood cells) contain a relatively high percentage of SOD. SOD helps rejuvenate the body cells by ensuring that harmful oxygen compounds such as the superoxide radical that develops during the respiration and metabolic process—and which can attack and destroy cells because of its oxidative power—are neutralized.[54] The normal superoxide radical content in the blood has an average value of 60 milliliter of blood. Even half of the average value is considered lethal since an uncontrolled superoxide radical leads to muscle deterioration, premature aging, cancer, arthritis, and other ailments.

SOD, a Cancer-Curing Remedy?

Physicians state that the therapeutic possibilities of SOD are breathtaking because we have a system of enzymes in reach in front of us that can slow down the aging process and prevent or reverse a long list of degenerative diseases. SOD is therefore also being increasingly discussed as a cancer-curing remedy. This enzyme complex is capable of neutralizing and rendering harmless cancer-causing substances like benzyprene (found in cigarette smoke) and the substances Try-P1 and Try-P2, residue from barbecued fish and meat. Dr. Yoshihide Hagiwara discovered (see his book on barley grass) that a water-soluble protein contained in SOD prevents the formation and multiplication of cancer cells that had been injected into mice. SOD also protects us against the effects of radioactive radiation. Even at an intensive rate of radiation (10,000 units of gamma radiation), the death rate of test animals was significantly reduced. SOD has also been used in the USA against the growth of tumors in the brain.[55]

The enzyme complex SOD is not only a potent radical-catcher but also famous for its detoxifying effects. Green barley grass juice and its extract can allow the body to eliminate many toxic substances that could otherwise accumulate and cause health disorders.

In addition, superoxide dismutase functions as a neurotransmitter (transmits nerve impulses between the brain and the nerves) and thereby promotes mental and physical fitness and agility. Nutrition experts especially recommend chewing the fresh, living grass because it delivers healing green living-cell food in the highest concentration.

Brain performance has been shown to be increased by the supplementation of glutaminic acid, a known neutrotransmitter. Glutaminic acid is successfully administered against senility, learning difficulties, and concentration disorders. In addition to barley grass, it can also be found in blue-green algae and kamut, the Egyptian primal wheat grass.[56] Glutaminic acid can therefore be called the "super fuel for the brain"; like SOD, it is capable of remedying symptoms of mental fatigue. Barley grass is therefore a "necessity" for students of all types and creative individuals who must achieve the highest level of mental performance.

The SOD in Barley Grass Against Toxins

It is interesting to note that barley and rice plants cannot be destroyed by the herbicide Paraquat because they both contain large amounts of SOD. Dr. Yoshihide Hagiwara calls SOD a "wonder remedy" because it protects cells from deterioration and the DNA in the cells from destruction.

SOD can only develop its activities when there are enough minerals like zinc or copper available.

For purifying the blood and lymph vessels, experts recommend drinking the following four times a day: four ounces of barley grass juice with the addition of 16 ounces of spring water to each glass for eliminating the toxins and deposits from all the organs. It is said that this therapy strengthens the immune system, has a blood-building effect, regenerates the cells, and has a lasting rejuvenating effect in the entire body, and especially for the skin.

Restoring the Acid-Alkaline Balance with Barley Grass Juice

Hyperacidity or "acidosis" is becoming one of the biggest health problems in the industrial nations. Our forests and soil are becoming increasingly "acidic," and this also has a correlation in our bodies. Because of diets with many products made of white flour, sweets, meat, milk products, and fish, we store increasingly more acids in our bodies. This effect is intensified by the use of stimulants such as coffee, black tea, and alcohol, as well as being aggravated by stress and a lack of rest periods in our output-oriented, restless society.

Instead of sleeping, resting, or meditating (a one-hour Reiki treatment moves the pH level up one point in the direction of alkaline) when they are exhausted in order to eliminate the collected acids and restore the acid-alkaline equilibrium, most people "dope" themselves with stimulants like sweets, cola drinks, caffeine-containing drinks, coffee, and black tea. As a result, they fall even further into the "red zone," into the acidic state of the body fluids. Consequently, they continually "overdraw" their "account." The body cells can no longer be energetically charged by this "excitant" effect, so the energy decrease that the person soon experiences demands another cola, coffee, or tea. Even routinely drinking two cups of coffee or black tea every day leads to a caffeine addiction. Any indoor plant watered with cola will die an acidic death within 48 hours. I've tested this myself! Above all, cola drinks are "poison" for children since the phosphoric acid that they contain decalcifies the bones and can even lead to osteoporosis in eleven-year-old children. Herbal teas, mineral water, and green tea are alternatives because the body metabolizes them as alkaline.

Cancer, Diabetes, and Rheumatism

Many diseases like diabetes, rheumatism, and cancer only "thrive" in acidic "soil." If we bring our bodies back to an acid-alkaline balance by eating alkaline foods such as fruit and vegetables or green juices, we take the acidic "soil" away from many diseases; as a result, our emotions are no longer "sour," but cheerful, relaxed, and optimistic.

In my book *Healing Power of Papaya*, there is an extensive chapter on "Help Against Acidosis (Hyperacidity)." In Germany, I give acidosis-therapy treatments in accordance with Dr. Renate Collier, as well as seminars (in the USA by request) in which I teach a massage technique for deacidifying the connective tissue, which is the acid-storage area of the body.

On the acid-alkaline scale, foods such as fish, meat, cheese spread, boiled eggs, roasted nuts, and white rice have the worst values, meaning that they form the most acid. Fresh olives, papaya, black radish, the leaves of red beets, blue-green (AFA) algae powder and algae, as well as barley grass and wheat grass, have the best values.[57] Our diets should consist from 70 to 80% of foods with high alkaline values and only 20 to 30% with acidic values. Most people have a diet with the reverse ratios! If you don't like black radish, fresh olives, or red beet leaves, then barley grass tablets or barley grass (fresh or mixed with water as a powder) is a wonderful alternative for "buffering" acids and avoiding an excess of acids, which leads to deposits and acidosis damage.

Dr. Mary Ruth Swope and Dr. Yoshihide Hagiwara consider barley grass and its extract to be the most alkaline food that we have. Dr. Yoshihide Hagiwara believes that barley grass is the king of all alkaline-forming foods. He considers green barley to be the best food for re-establishing an acid-alkaline balance in the body. Spinach, one of the other foods that forms alkaline, has a value of 39.6 (milligrams of alkaline material present in 100 grams) on his table, while Green Magma achieves a value of 66.4. It far exceeds other alkaline-formers such as bananas (7.9), tomatoes (5.6), oranges (4.5), and lettuce (3.8).[58] No wonder that barley grass extract is such a potent alkaline-forming remedy since it overshadows all of the vegetables, fruit, and other types of grains studied in terms of the minerals it contains. Dr. Yoshihide Hagiwara claims that green barley essence (Green Magma) supplies a larger amount and a better balance of minerals than any other food that is generally valued for the health of its nutrients.

Dr. Mary Ruth Swope also discusses the alkalizing effect of barley grass. The most frequent signs of an acid-alkaline imbalance are heart pains, exhaustion, dry skin, breathlessness, irritability, sleep disorders, hard stools, restlessness, and brittle fingernails. With test strips (pharmacy), it is easily possible for us to find the pH value of our urine or saliva. However, Dr. Mary Ruth Swope absolutely does not recommend taking alkaline preparations since these are inorganic minerals and this approach is a "cover-up" method and not a causal therapy. She concludes that dried barley grass juice is an excellent source of alkaline in order to somewhat counteract our acid-forming diets. In her opinion, this effect truly makes it a food with true power.

Unborn Children Profit from Barley Grass Juice

Nutrition experts also emphasize the intensely deacidifying effect of barley grass through its ample alkaline minerals and trace elements. Fresh grass juices and grass extracts in raw-food quality can also heal the cause of the wide-spread disease of hyperacidity. All gland functions, as well as the production of hydrochloric acid, are dependent upon the pH value; this means that they only function optimally in an acid-alkaline balance. Enzymes, including those responsible for metabolism and digestion, as well as thought processes and every other vital process, only act within a specific pH range. Many enzymes slow down or completely stop their activities when the environment becomes too acidic. Incidentally, barley grass juice has the same pH value as breast milk. They therefore recommend raising small children who have been weaned on barley grass juice, green juices, and green plant food so that they achieve their optimal physical and mental level of development.

Even during pregnancy, the mother-to-be should be sure to eat a diet with high alkaline values. Dr. Yoshihide Hagiwara discovered that women who were conscious of their acid-alkaline balance, including the use of barley grass juice, during their pregnancies, also gave birth to healthy, emotionally well-balanced, and cheerful children. However, the expectant mothers who did not eat enough alkaline-forming foods and instead consumed an acid-forming diet were more likely to give birth to children with a weak constitution and imbalanced moods. Children who are given an improper diet tend to become overly sensitive and impatient, and many of them develop abnormal motor behavior.

Today, many children are quick to become irritable, whiny, and hyperactive. Could the cause for this be found in an acid-forming diet while they were still in the womb? The mother provides the "soil" for the fetus to grow in, which is why a balanced diet rich in vital substances is extremely important during pregnancy for healthy development of the fruit of the womb.

Barley Grass Juice, a Rejuvenating Elixir

Enzymes in Barley Grass Repair Damaged Cells

I can't promise you that you will become immortal with barley grass juice. But barley grass juice can help you to rejuvenate aging cells, slow down the aging process, and give you the feeling of being more vital and lively.

Grass juices are full of enzymes and improve the blood picture. Viktoras Kulvinskas believes that there is no quicker, safer way of regulating digestion and providing the cells with nutrition than the intake of chlorophyll.[59] Dr. Weston Price, founder of the Price-Pottenger Nutrition Foundation, isolated one substance from the tips of young grasses that promotes the regeneration of damaged cells. Young cereal grasses can therefore be used as a rejuvenation tonic. Barley grass juice detoxified the body because chlorophyll promotes the elimination of mucous, crystallized acids, and other waste materials; furthermore, it supports good digestion. Fifteen pounds of wheat grass or barley grass correspond approximately to the nutritional value of 350 pounds (!) of organically grown vegetables.

Dr. Ann Wigmore, in her book called *Be Your Own Doctor*, (see Bibliography on page 147) writes that experts have isolated more than one-hundred substances, including all of the known minerals, from barley grass and wheat grass. On the eighth day of growth, cereal grass that has been grown on the windowsill contains all of the essential amino acids. Wheat grass or barley grass can therefore be considered a truly complete food.

With their balanced nutrient profile, cereal grasses optimally provide undernourished body cells with all the essential amino acids, vitamins, and minerals, as well as stimulating the rate of cell division. Barley grass is the richest natural source of SOD (also see previous chapter in this book on page 94 ff.); it is not only a cancer-inhibiting enzyme, but as an extraordinarily effective free-radical catcher it also possesses the ability of reducing the cell-decomposing oxidative force in the body. When the cells are receiving a poor supply of SOD, they lose the ability of renewing themselves and die prematurely.

SOD plays an important role by slowing down certain aging processes or even preventing them. Experts discovered that the aging process takes place more quickly under the condition of a low SOD level. Gerontologists have determined that short-lived fruit flies have low SOD values while fruit flies with a longer life span have high SOD values.

SOD Protection Is Important

Scientists who research the possibilities for extending life are increasingly studying SOD. Dr. Hans Kugler, author of *Slowing Down the Aging Process* and *Seven Keys to a Longer Life*, is particularly interested in the center of the brain that controls the aging process. He believes that imbalances of the neurotransmitters, meaning the chemical substances through which our nerve cells communicate with each other, can mean everything from accelerated aging to depression or other mental disorders. One component that is a key to this process is the neurotransmitter norepinephrine, which is very quickly destroyed by the presence of the superoxide radical. The destruction of just just a small percentage of the norephinephrine accelerates the aging process and leads to depressions. This is why it is so important to be protected by SOD.[60] As a result of animal experiments, scientists have discovered that a large amount of SOD can double the life span of laboratory animals.

The nucleic acids consumed in the diet may also promote the formation of repair of DNA and RNA, the genetic component of our cells.

Barley Grass Rejuvenates the Cells and Skin

Green juices from cultivated grasses are affordable for anyone. They are a living-cell treatment without any side effects, stimulating the renewal of the cells in a natural manner through specific growth factors. The blue pigment phycocyanin contained in barley grass, as well as chlorophyll, iron, and vitamin B, stimulate the bone marrow and contribute to the formation of red and white blood cells.

Fitness and mental alertness, as well as joy in life and élan, depend on the energy supply through living foods, as well as the quick and smooth digestion of our food. Halima Neumann believes that the only natural aid for increasing the digestibility of the food and the speed in which decomposition products are efficiently brought to elimination is non-heated plant green—the key to the fountain of youth.

In addition to barley grass, other foods can be recommended as "rejuvenation elixirs": blue-green algae, raw spinach (disadvantage: high proportion of oxalic acid), alfalfa sprouts, and fresh comfrey leaves. Alfalfa can easily be raised on the windowsill, but it can also be purchased as a powder or tablets; comfrey, which is also healthy in large amounts (despite prejudice against it), makes no special demands as it grows on the balcony or in the garden.

Proteins are considered the "building blocks of life" and are important for cell renewal. Barley grass powder consists of up to about 45% protein, which therefore is the largest individual component. In comparison, wheat flour only contains 10% protein. Barley grass juice contains an especially large amount of the light protein molecules or peptides, which can be used in a very simple manner by the body. Barley grass juice has all of the essential amino acids in an easily digestible form and in such proportions that the body can use it to build optimal tissue. Among other things, analyses show that barley grass contains the essential amino acids valine, leucine, isoleucine, phenylalanine, and methionine in a stable state.

In contrast to wheat grass, the abundant amount of glutaminic acid improves the short-term and long-term memory, increases the speed of reactions, improves learning ability, and serves as Alzheimer's prevention.[61] There are about 250 mg of glutaminic acid per 10 g of barley grass powder.

The skin is considered the mirror of our health. Rough or inflamed skin frequently indicates problems in the stomach and intestinal area, a swollen face can be a sign for liver or kidney problems; pimples and blackheads are a sign of hyperacidity and the accumulation of waste materials in the body. Because of its abundance of minerals, enzymes, and vitamins, barley grass juice is capable of rejuvenating the cells of the inner organs and skin. The therapy with grass juice strengthens the immune system, has a blood-building effect, regenerates the cells, and causes a lasting rejuvenation effect in the entire body, but especially in the skin. The effect of green barley grass extract for rejuvenating the skin has been confirmed in clinical studies carried out by Dr. Tatsuo Muto (see note 15).

The substances in barley grass are capable of stopping the growth of cancer cells; they enable the body to eliminate toxins that would otherwise continue to accumulate and lead to chronic diseases and premature aging.

Barley Grass Helps You Feel Full of Energy, No Matter What Your Age!

In her book on barley grass, Dr. Mary Ruth Swope includes reports on the experiences of people who are convinced that they are giving their body cells the necessary nutrients for moving body and mind in the direction of health, youthfulness, and abundant energy when they take the barley grass extract.

Here are a few statements from readers about her book: "I feel that green barley grass extract has restored my vitality. I'm waiting to see what the new doctor, I'm moving soon, says about a leukemia patient who radiates so much vital energy." "Since I had severe bronchitis, I have been constantly exhausted. Now I can once again work for hours without a break, and because I look so good, people ask how I do it." "I tried barley grass powder because I was constantly tired and listless. Now I constantly have a feeling of energy and well-being. You value something like this more when you've had to be without it for so long. It must be the barley grass because I haven't changed anything else in my life." "As an alcoholic, I had already been dry for 14 months. After taking barley grass powder for just three weeks, I no longer had any headaches; but, even better: I got back my joy and optimism and my memory has improved considerably."

Barley Grass Against Radioactivity and Cell Damage

Barley grass represents a great aid in the atomic age. Throughout the world, there are more than 500 nuclear power plants and a number of reprocessing plants in operation that increase the damage caused by radioactivity. Even television sets "bombard" us with cell-destroying radiation. It is therefore important to sit at least twelve feet away from the television set and consciously limit our viewing time.

Radiation is damaging to the cells at any dosage, even low-level continual radiation. At higher levels or continual radiation, radioactivity kills cells. The rate of leukemia rises, especially for children, in areas close to nuclear power plants. In addition, there is also the strain of radiation through x-rays such as during mammograms.

"There are numerous scientific studies that prove the value of green barley grass in supporting the cells that have been damaged by radioactivity." (DR. MARY RUTH SWOPE IN *"GREEN LEAVES OF BARLEY"*)

When I recently went to the dentist and he couldn't find any problem despite the fact that the last visit had been four-and-a-half years (!) earlier (which I attribute to my healthy diet and daily Reiki treatments), he wanted to x-ray my teeth. His reason: "After four-and-a-half years, there *must* be something wrong!" I didn't have any complaints. Many physicians are apparently careless in their use of this diagnostic technique, which is always a burden on the body; perhaps, this is because they need to pay off their expensive equipment.

The damage through UV radiation is also increasing. Despite prohibition of chlorofluorocarbons, which destroy the ozone layer, it will take at least 20 years for this natural protection from the sun to regenerate itself. Because of the increased UV radiation, leading dermatologists predict a doubling of the melonoma within the next ten years.

Drink Barley Grass Before and After X-Rays!

It certainly doesn't make sense to worry about the negative effects of radioactivity because worries and fears additionally weaken our immune system. We can thank God that barley grass juice and wheat grass juice are outstanding remedies for protecting ourselves against the effects of radioactivity and even regenerating tissue that has been damaged by radioactivity. It has been determined that chlorophyll increases the resistance to radioactivity. In an experiment with guinea pigs, all of which received a deadly dosage of x-rays, 97% of those fed with the customary food died within twenty days; 44% of those fed with carrots died as well, but none of the guinea pigs who were fed dark-green vegetables.

The chlorophyll in barley grass may help promote the formation of new blood cells—also see the chapter on "Chlorophyll, the Blood of Plants" on page 15 ff. and "The Healing Effects of Barley Grass" on page 89 ff. in this book. Barley grass juice accelerates the formation of cells. By drinking barley grass or wheat grass juice, the development of the lactase required for digestion is promoted, which also diminished the damage from radioactivity. It is therefore important to drink barley grass juice before and after x-rays are taken in order to protect ourselves against damage from radioactivity!

The enzymes in barley grass help in the renewal of radiation-damaged carriers of genetic information (DNA) and fighting the cell-damaging free radicals that are produced in any type of radiation exposure (for example, from watching television, x-rays, irradiated food, microwave ovens, and nuclear radiation). Food heated in microwaves, which is a common practice in fast-food restaurants and American homes, contains unnatural and harmful substances. Directly after food prepared in microwave ovens is eaten, it is possible to observe changes in the blood similar to the triggering of a cancer process.[62]

Dr. Mary Ruth Swope says that enzymes such as SOD, glutamine peroxidase, methionine reductase, and catalase (all of which are present in barley grass juice) are potent antioxidants. She also believes that our body mainly uses them in the first line of defense to fight the free radicals produced by radiation. They are nature's true healing remedy for us. Through his research, Dr. Yoshihide Hagiwara discovered that the abundance of enzymes of barley grass juice and lecithin-like substances can restore and repair DNA that has been exposed to radioactivity or environmental radiation.

Ronald L. Seibold claims that there is not yet a complete explanation of how green foods like barley grass juice protect us against chemical carcinogens (cancer-causing substances) and radiation. Apparently, chlorophyll, beta carotene, and vitamin C play a special role in this process. The protein P4D1, which is amply present in barley grass, stimulates repair of the DNA, including the reproductive cells. Dr. Mary Ruth Swope therefore surmises that this protein may prevent deformations in newborn babies. According to experts, about two glasses of barley grass juice a day are enough to neutralize the radioactive stress to which people living in large cities are currently subjected.

Heavy Metals Can Be Eliminated with Barley Grass Juice!

With its abundance of enzymes, including the super free-radical catcher SOD, barley grass juice also helps protect us against the cell-destroying effects of UV light. Moreover, it can even heal existing cell damage. This helps us prevent the development of the black melanoma, a particularly insidious type of cancer. In addition to barley grass and wheat grass, according to Dr. Taussig of the University of Hawaii, bromelain also protects against UV radiation and the development of skin cancer in dosages starting at 500 mg. This problem appears to be increasingly dangerous.

Besides taking barley grass juice for its cell-protecting vitamins and valuable enzyme complexes on a daily basis, it also is important for strengthening the immune system (especially for people who live in large cities) in view of the increasing radiation stress. The consumption of denatured, heated food and poisons like alcohol and nicotine should be limited; on the other hand, it is important to gradually increase the amount of living, unheated food that is rich in enzymes, vitamins, and minerals up to about 80% of the diet. The glutamic acid contained in barley grass reduces the desire for harmful substances like alcohol, coffee, nicotine, sweets, and drugs. As a result, it has made a name for itself in the USA as a remedy for fighting addictions.

Barley grass is also very helpful in removing harmful heavy metals such as lead, which can lead to learning and behavior disorders, especially in children. Its proportions of trace elements such as zinc, copper, and selenium promote the detoxification. Through the high content of beta carotene and chlorophyll, the metabolic processes in the liver are supported, which also relieves, strengthens, and detoxifies the liver. (Blue-green algae has a similar effect.)

Barley Grass Against Cancer

Most Types of Cancer
Will Double within 20 Years!

The World Health Organization (WHO) predicts that most types of cancer will double their rates within the next twenty years. The developing nations are copying the unhealthy lifestyles prevailing in the industrial nations: much denatured food, large amounts of meat and dairy products, and too much fast food, sugar, and fat, but too little fruit and vegetables. As a result the rate of cancer in these developing countries is also rising.

I work as a developmental-aid volunteer in Haiti, one of the poorest countries in the Western Hemisphere. During my visits there, I have seen how healthy foods such as whole-grain manioc bread is being displaced by imported white flour; young Haitians, in particular, are just "wild" about cola drinks, sugared condensed milk, hot dogs, chocolate, cigarettes, and junk food.

Not just avoiding causes of cancer, but also cancer therapy appears to create major problems. Physician Dr. Mary Ruth Swope criticizes that chemotherapy is not as effective as it is frequently depicted. Studies clearly show that this therapy only has limited success in lengthening the life of the afflicted person. While the actual cancer cells in the blood are destroyed, healthy cells are also attacked and the immune system weakened by chemotherapy. In addition, chemotherapy has the effect of causing cancer cells to grow stronger in order to successfully combat the "attacking" medication. Dr. Mary Ruth Swope believes that when Americans want to be cured of cancer, heart diseases, arthritis, diabetes, obesity, and a vast quantity of factors that weaken them, they must find unconventional treatment methods containing nutrition and other healing remedies that nature provides as their main components.

Many physicians worldwide have also recognized that the victory over cancer can only take place through the healing power of the body with a strong immune system but cannot function through immuno-suppressive methods. Professor Wagner of the Institute for Pharmaceutical Biology at the University of Munich is researching the phenomenon of "spontaneous healing," meaning what conditions lead to people becoming cured "overnight" on their own of such serious diseases as cancer.

Barley Grass Strengthens the Immune System

Taking barley grass on a regular basis strengthens our immune system and enables it to successfully fight cancer cells. Our bodies produce about 5,000 to 10,000 cancer cells every day. A healthy body with a strong, effective immune system is capable of successfully fighting these cancer cells and eliminating them. Barley grass amply provides all of the nutrients necessary for the production of immune cells in a balanced form. We should naturally not only strengthen our immune system through barley grass juice but also through a healthy diet with a large proportion of fresh fruits and vegetables. Furthermore, exercise in the fresh air and a relaxation technique practiced on a regular basis, such as the authentic Reiki®, affords deep relaxation and reduction of stress.

WHO predicts that most types of cancer will double within 20 years

Cooked foods promote the growth of cancer cells, while raw foods let cancer cells shrink. In my health handbook *Healing Power of Papaya*, (see Bibliography page 147) there is documentation from extensive literature on the healing success with raw foods. Dr. Max Gerson, a friend of the famous physician Albert Schweitzer, also became well-known for his success in healing cancer patients rejected for further treatment by conventional medicine by giving them a diet consisting mainly of freshly squeezed green juices and fruit juices from organically grown fruits and vegetables. This is extensively documented in his book *A Cancer Therapy: Results of Fifty Cases and the Cure of Advanced Cancer* (see Bibliography page 146).

Barley grass cleanses the digestive system and supports the healthy formation of blood so that the cells are first detoxified and then abundantly provided with the urgently necessary nutrients. Substantial portions of our immune system are located in the intestines. Barley grass extract, which is rich in roughage, is especially helpful in the prevention of intestinal cancer, a type of cancer that is the second most frequently occurring in the USA. The fibers of green plants allow the chyme to pass through the intestines more quickly.

Through its strongly alkaline effect, barley grass juice changes the body environment. Many diseases such as rheumatism and cancer can only grow in an excessively acidic environment, "acidic soil." Cancer patients always have an acidosis, a hyperacidity of the body fluids, especially around the cancer cells, with an extremely acidic pH value of 5.5 to 6. Barley grass is one of the most potent, if not *the* most potent, food for restoring an acid-alkaline balance without any side-effects like those of the alkali preparations.

The Antioxidants
Against Cell Damage

Barley grass contains many antioxidants such as vitamin C, E, provitamin A, and selenium, which have been proved to be capable of fighting free radicals (aggressive oxygen compounds that contribute to the development of cancer). These free-radical-catchers and "anticancer vitamins" are also used in supportive cancer therapy. Barley grass juice contains about twice as much beta carotene as carrots, and the carotene in dark vegetables is converted into vitamin A twice as effectively as that in carrots.

Dark-green vegetables with a high content of beta carotene can give smokers a certain amount of protection against lung cancer. Eating green vegetables such as barley grass or broccoli reduces the risk of contracting certain diseases like ovarian cancer, throat cancer, skin cancer, lung cancer, or stomach cancer. In general, older people who eat large amounts of green and yellow vegetables are far less likely to die of cancer.[63]

Many members of the medical profession feel that the widespread lack of selenium in our soil and blood serum is contributing to the increase of cancer diseases. Selenium protects us against harmful free radicals and environmental toxins like cadmium, lead, and nitrites: it is abundantly present in barley grass.

Certain enzymes in barley grass such as peroxidase, catalase, and superoxide dismutase (SOD) are capable of repairing and regenerating the damaged DNA in the cell nucleus caused by radioactivity, for example. This also includes the reproductive organs. The enzyme, SOD can apparently prevent the formation of cancer cells. According to studies by Professor T. Horio of Japan, barley grass juice is apparently capable of weakening the mutation-producing effect of the cancer-causing substances in grilled meat and fish.

According to studies at the University of Texas System Cancer Center in Houston, chlorophyll, which is amply present in barley grass, inhibits the metabolism of carcinogens. This discovery was made by Dr. Chui Nan Lai. Many scientific studies have confirmed that chlorophyll reduces the ability of carcinogens to cause gene mutations. Chlorophyll-rich plant extracts neutralize the cancer-causing effect of charcoal dust, tobacco smoke, barbecued meat, and red wine. Ronald L. Seibold states that in this capacity, chlorophyllin (a water solution of a chlorophyll derivative) is more effective against mutations triggered by the above-mentioned mixtures than vitamin A, vitamin C, or vitamin E.

The passage of food through the intestines is accelerated by dietary fiber or roughage, which is amply present in most barley grass powders. As a result, cancer-causing substances do not have a long exposure time in the sensitive intestinal mucosa. In particular, this prevents the development of colon cancer, hemorrhoids, and irritable colon. The American Cancer Society and the National Cancer Institute therefore recommend generous consumption of dietary fiber.

Barley Grass Against Cancer Cells

With respect to cancer, barley grass has a preventive, as well as a healing effect. Dr. Yoshihide Hagiwara has determined that when mice with cancer were fed barley grass extract, they experienced a much higher rate of recovery than the control group. He discovered that a water-soluble protein contained in the SOD enzyme complex develops this anti-cancer effect and is capable of suppressing the development of cancer cells. Another protein, peridoxase, can apparently render the cancer-causing substances Try-P1 and Try-P2 harmless.[64] Another enzyme that is significant for cancer therapy is catalase. Catalase is capable of decomposing hydrogen peroxide (H_2O_2) into water and oxygen, making it harmless in the process. Hydrogen peroxide is produced during respiration and has a toxic and cell-destroying effect in the body.

Milk and dairy products reduce the activity of catalase because they lack the necessary minerals copper and iron, which are richly present in barley grass. Other foods such as bread from white flour, polished rice, and butter—which also hardly contain any copper and iron—can apparently hinder the activity of certain important enzymes in the body and therefore contribute to the development of cancer. Dr. Yoshihide Hagiwara believes that the key to preventing cancer can be found here.

Its high proportion of mucopolysaccharides is also apparently responsible for the cancer-preventing effect of barley grass. It has been proved that the mucopolysaccharides in shiitake mushrooms (fomes glaucotos) and in bamboo grass have anti-carcinogenic qualities. These substances can be found in barley grass in even larger concentrations than in these foods.

Barley Grass Can Heal Destroyed Genes

Dr. Yoshihide Hagiwara reports on American scientific studies in which the DNA genes destroyed by cancer were regenerated into healthy genes when green barley grass juice was used. In the books by Dr. Mary Ruth Swope and Dr. Yoshihide Hagiwara, there are many reports on the experiences of people with cancer who had their health disorders either improved or cured by taking barley grass juice. Barley grass extract contains an abundance of enzymes and lecithin-like substances. These engage in complex activities, repair the DNA, and completely restore the DNA that has mutated through x-rays or environmental toxins.

A type of vitamin E has been discovered in barley grass, alpha-tocopherol succinate. It has been demonstrated that this vitamin protects against colon cancer and breast cancer. It prevents the reproduction of cancer cells ten times more effectively than the other type of vitamin E, alpha-tocoperol.

Another component of barley grass with cancer-preventing and cancer-destroying effects has been identified by Dr. Allan Goldstein (from the George Washington University in Washington D.C.); however, when this book was written he did not yet have a name for it and called it the "mysterious molecule." Perhaps I will have the opportunity to inform you about it in a second volume.

The actual goal of medicine should be to protect people against illness and look after their physical and emotional well-being. Preventive medicine has been neglected up to now, and this situation has worsened due to economy measures in the health field. As a result, we are all called upon to take responsibility for our own health and let go of this consumer attitude: "I'm paying for health insurance, and that's enough." The daily consumption of green vegetables or barley grass juice can be a step in the right direction of assuming more personal responsibility in taking care of our own health and preventing cancer.

Healthy with Just Barley Grass Juice?

—The Broader Perspective—

Contentment and Fulfillment in Our Working and Private Lives

"For the Kingdom of God does not mean food and drink but righteousness and peace and joy in the Holy Spirit." (ROMANS 14:17)

Is it enough to just change our diets and give barley grass a permanent place on the menu? Unfortunately, it is not. Healthy food rich in vital substances is merely one factor, but possibly even the most important factor, required for radiant health. Other significant aspects are physical activity, adequate rest and relaxation, much fresh air, and moderate but daily absorption of the sun's energy.

A very effective method for deep relaxation and reduction of stress is the authentic Reiki®, a method for activating the universal energy. (I teach this method worldwide in seminars.) We do not live from bread alone—from what we have on our plate or in our glass—but are "nourished" by many, many other things!

Satisfying personal and social relationships are important for our health, as well as work that is fulfilling and makes us content. Many suggestions for developing the necessary self-confidence for this step can be found in Deepak Chopra's book on *The Seven Spiritual Laws of Success* (see Bibliography on page 146)

Exercise in the fresh air on a regular basis is important for stimulating all of the metabolic processes, for an optimal supply of oxygen to our cells, for a strong and stress-resistant heart, for the reduction of stress—and even as a preventive, and for eliminating waste materials from the body. The lymphatic fluid, which is responsible for transporting waste materials such as harmful viruses and bacteria from the cellular metabolism to the eliminatory organs, is dependent upon muscle contractions. The cells stay healthy through movement! Half an hour of fast walking, jogging, or jumping on the trampoline every day—outside, if possible—is enough to stimulate our lymph nodes and keep the lymphatic fluid moving. I jog for at least half an hour every day, no matter what the weather. In addition, I have a children's trampoline that we use on a regular basis. This also keeps our lymphatic system moving. If you aren't doing it yet, start a program of endurance training for half-an-hour at least three times a week. You will feel the difference in your level of joy and energy!

A Healthy Mind in a Healthy Body

Mental and emotional problems such as addictions can also be caused by a poor state of physical health. Is a lack of energy or weak drive perhaps less a symptom than the cause for problems like drug abuse, overweight, or depression? Dr. Ann Wigmore was one of the first to discover that young people can be freed from drug addiction through a diet rich in vital substances, with a large proportion of cereal juices. In any case, barley grass juice with all of its nutrients is a good possibility for raising our energy level and achieving a more positive, optimistic attitude. This can allow us to break out of the vicious circle of conditions like depression and bad health. With the help of barley grass, we can move in a spiral of continually escalating well-being of body and mind, which intensifies itself through the positive mental attitude that increasingly leads us to what is truly good for us.

It is also important to know our true needs (and this book is also intended for this purpose) and "nourish" ourselves increasingly with the best of everything that life has to offer: "Love your neighbor *as yourself.*" We nourish ourselves not only with food, water, and oxygen but also by giving and receiving love and advancing our personal growth. Mother Meera answered the question "what is sin?" in the following manner: "there is only one sin, and that is not loving enough."[65]

Our own health and our fulfilled, happy life is not just something that is important to us alone; it is also important for everyone else. Imagine a world in which everyone was radiantly healthy, fulfilled, and happy! Perhaps we can become an example for our fellow human beings, who are often unknowing and therefore without orientation.

Green is the color of life, hope, renewal, and growth. In order to connect and nourish ourselves with these energies, it is important to have an appropriate amount of green food in our diet. Our surrounding world is also full of the green force that we can simply become more aware of: plants give us life-providing oxygen, and every spring reminds us of the power of life, no matter how long and hard the previous winter may have been. By absorbing the color green, we connect with the nature inside of us and around us.

Mixing green juices is so simple that we all have a few minutes a day to do it. It is important for us to nourish ourselves with the best possible food on all levels. Take the necessary steps in your life to more health for the body, mind, and soul. If you do this, I thank you for the inspiration you are to all of us. If you have not yet achieved your full potential of health and joy in life, then simply eat more green foods! If this book has inspired you, then its goal has been fulfilled. In addition, may this book express a small part of the ascending spirals of planetary consciousness that is preparing us for a quantum leap of recognizing the unity of all people on this planet and their oneness with the divine.

Recipes with Barley Grass

All types of juices from vegetables and sprouts can be mixed with barley grass juice or wheat grass juice and diluted with spring water (revitalizing) or water with a low level of carbonation. White grape juice, pear juice, apricot juice, and juice from blueberries or papayas also mix well with it. Or dilute apple sauce (from organic cultivation, if possible) and naturally without added sugar (health food store or natural food store). Grapes strengthen the function of the gallbladder and liver. Acidic juices like grapefruit juice or lemon juice are not appropriate since the acid causes the living enzymes in the barley grass juice to quickly stop their activities. Barley grass powder can also be stirred into the above-mentioned juices.

Barley grass also tastes very good stirred into soy milk or rice milk. Or mix it with sweet whey powder with a vanilla taste.

The recommended dosage of barley grass powder is to take between two teaspoons and one tablespoon, which is from 5 to 10 g, with 6 to 7 ounces of non-acidic liquid three times a day about one-half hour before meals. Do not eat any solid food for about twenty minutes after taking it. In the morning, a barley grass drink mobilizes the deacidification of the body and removal of its waste materials. In the evening, a barley grass meal, either liquid or solid, supports restful sleep because the acid content of the blood is reduced. Also, tryptophan (a neurotransmitter that is converted into serotinin by the body), of which 11 to 15 mg are contained in 10 g of barley grass powder, makes it easy to fall asleep and sleep restfully. Besides in barley grass, tryptophan is also present in avocados, pineapples, bananas, almonds, sesame, and spinach. However, heat above 50 degrees C destroys it.

When two to three tablespoons of grass powder are mixed with clear vegetable soup, vegetable juices, rice or almond milk, soy or diluted coconut milk, this replaces a complete meal. When I do this, I feel satisfied for hours afterward and am mentally alert and lively. When traveling, I always have a jar of gently pressed barley grass tablets with me. These help keep me feeling alert. When I am stuck in traffic, the barley tablets help my body neutralize the exhaust fumes. All grass juices increase the powers of resistance, even against radioactivity and x-rays. They also help eliminate heavy metal from the body. Always eat with liquids!

Healing Fasts with Barley Grass

Barley grass is low in fat, but it does have a large amount of dietary fiber and just 29 calories per 100 g. This makes it the ideal natural food substitute for overweight people who want to reduce excess protein and fat. In warm liquids, barley grass powder is very satisfying and expands greatly. It is therefore ideal for use in healing fasts. As an alternative, freshly squeezed barley grass juice can be used—or mix it with the powder! A 30-gram portion of barley grass powder, which corresponds to three tablespoons, should be mixed with 500 ml of liquids. It replaces a complete meal. Barley grass powder can also be mixed well with blue-green algae powder.

Healing crises are soothed when fasting with barley grass; waste materials and acids are eliminated more quickly with it. Fresh green juices from cultivated grasses or, as an alternative, grass in powder form are also one of the best lymph-cleansing agents. It allows us to remain charged with energy and in a good mood. While fasting, an individual should be sure that the intestines are cleansed every morning. Take either magnesium sulfate (Epsom salt from the pharmacy, one teaspoon to approx. eight ounces of lukewarm water) or one tablespoon of psyllium husks to eight ounces of water so that there is no recurring toxification through the intestinal wall and encrusted waste substances can be dissolved from the intestinal villi.

The content of more than 20% easily digestible protein ensures a safe healing or partial fast with barley grass, optimally providing the nerves and brain with nutrients. With its choline, the complete vitamin-B "family" present in this grass juice guarantees a stabile acetylcholine level and consequently prevents nervousness, restlessness, and sleep disorders.

Barley Grass Beverages

Green Power

Stir one heaping teaspoon each of barley grass powder, blue-green algae powder, and kamut powder into a glass of purified and revitalized water or low-carbonation mineral water. Drink this power pick-me-up three times a day and whenever necessary; for example, if you are tired or have concentration problems. I add two teaspoons of psyillum husk to my morning drink to promote intestinal cleansing. The Green Magna barley grass powder also tastes deliciously nutlike when mixed in water with blue-green algae.

Green Smoothie

Put one apple or one papaya in the blender with two teaspoons of barley grass powder, or fresh barley grass juice, and one glass of low-carbonation water. Mix for about 30 seconds at the lowest speed. This juice contains much calcium, iron, magnesium, and high-quality protein.

Breakfast Smoothie

Take two bananas, one small apple, one teaspoon of barley grass powder, or freshly squeezed barley grass juice, and one glass of purified and energized water. Puree and mix everything at the second lowest speed for about 30 seconds. This breakfast makes us feel immediately fit and alert. It is the ideal brain and nerve food—and is filling for hours afterward! The color and taste are like slightly sweetened creamed spinach.

Tropical Energy Shake

Take two cups of pineapple in pieces, two cups of unfiltered apple juice, one small ripe banana, and two teaspoons of barley grass powder. Mix all of the ingredients in a blender. This shake contains many enzymes, minerals, and vitamins. It tastes delicious.

Anti-Stress and Anti-Acid Drink
(Based on a recipe by Halima Neumann)

Take three ounces of magnesium-rich dark-red berry juice from ripe blackberries, blueberries, or black currants. Juice in a blender (or buy the concentrated juices from the health food store). Add one tablespoon of blue-green algae powder and two tablespoons of barley grass powder. If you would like to reduce the fat in your body and aren't allergic to soy, add one tablespoon of soy-lecithin granulated powder. You can also add one to two tablespoons of almond-milk powder to strengthen your nerves and bones.

Kidney Cleansing and Strengthening Drink
(Based on a recipe by Halima Neumann)

Use one tablespoon of blue-green algae, two tablespoons of barley grass powder. Add ten ounces of the fruit water from a green coconut or sixteen ounces of watermelon juice or 500 g of melon fruit pulp. Juice everything in a blender and sieve the seeds.

A warm pumpkin-onion soup or green bean-onion soup can also be eaten in the evening to strengthen the kidneys: Let it cool to mouth temperature and stir in the blue-green algae and barley grass. Ginger, curcuma can also be added as seasoning.

Tomato Drink

Use one small celery stick, two medium-sized tomatoes, one teaspoon of barley grass powder, and one pinch of pepper. First process the celery in the juicer, then add the tomatoes and season with barley grass powder, pepper, and possibly one squirt of tamari (soy) sauce or 1/2 teaspoon of miso soy paste. This is good for removing fluids and waste substances from the body!

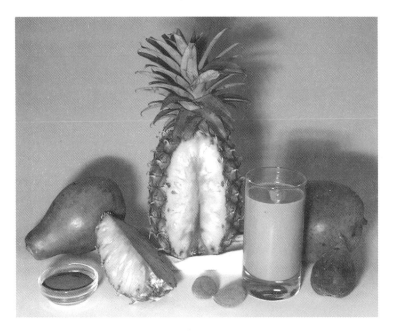

Fruit Drink

Take one-half of a fresh pineapple or one baby pineapple. Peel and cut into pieces. Add 60 g of fresh barley grass (or one tablespoon of barley grass powder) and three leaves of fresh mint or lemon balm. The pineapple can be juiced in a normal juicer and the barley grass in a berry or wheat-grass juicer. Mix with a small amount of water and decorate with mint or lemon balm leaves. This juice not only strengthens the spirits but also the libido.

Apple Dream

Take two medium-sized apples and 60 g of fresh barley grass. Cut the apples into small pieces, put them into a berry juicer, and add the barley grass juice. If you would like to have it sweeter, add a handful of seedless grapes at the end. This juice contains potassium, pectin, and glucose. It also removes excess fluids and detoxified the body. If you don't have any fresh barley grass, you can mix in one tablespoon of barley grass powder instead.

Power Drink

For this fitness drink, use three medium-sized organic carrots, 100 g of mixed sprouts or wild herbs, and 60 g of fresh barley grass (or one tablespoon barley grass powder). Juice the carrots in the juicer, and then add the sprouts or wild herbs and the barley grass powder into a berry juicer and juice. Mix all the ingredients and serve. Can be garnished with nasturtium, which can also be eaten. This power drink contains many enzymes and abundant provitamin A.

Red-Beet Fitness Drink

Take one small peeled red beet, one-half of a peeled cucumber cut into pieces, and 60 g of barley grass (or one tablespoon of barley grass powder). If the cucumber is organic, you can also use the peel. Cut the red beet into small pieces and juice the ingredients one at a time in the berry juicer. Add the barley grass last because it quickly oxidizes. Mix everything. This juice contains much iron (good for women during pregnancy and menstruation!) and potassium. Red beets are said to have a cancer-preventing and -healing effect.

Green Dream

Use three tablespoons of freshly squeezed barley grass juice (or one tablespoon of barley grass powder) for this juice. Add four ounces of freshly squeezed grape juice from light grapes, one tablespoon of herb tea (such as oregano or nettle), pepper or papaya pepper (from dried papaya seeds), and some herb salt. Mix all of the ingredients well. The juice even tastes good without salt and pepper!

Tropical Hawaiian Drink

To make this delicious juice, use four ounces freshly squeezed barley grass juice or juice from barley grass powder, pure mango juice, one tablespoon of honeydew melon juice, and mineral water.

Mix all of the juices well and fill with mineral water. If desired, add ice cubes and garnish with pineapple wedges.

Sauces for Salads and Dips

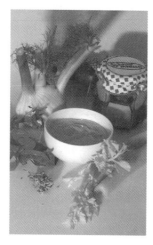

Basic Sauce Recipe

Use one heaping teaspoon of barley grass powder, 200 g of vegetables such as tomatoes, cucumbers, turnip, or zucchini, one handful of nori algae, one avocado, and six ounces of kombucha drink. First puree the hard vegetables with the algae and kombucha drink in the blender, then add the soft vegetables. Keep blending and add the barley grass powder. This sauce makes enough for four to six people. If you put it in an airtight jar in the refrigerator, it should stay fresh for a few days.

Barley Grass Sauce

This sauce contains only high-quality fats and lowers the cholesterol level (in comparison to many of the conventional sauces). Use four tablespoons of cold-pressed olive oil, sixteen ounces of barley grass juice, one chopped bayberry leaf, one pinch of herb salt, one teaspoon of yeast flakes, one pinch of stevia powder (to sweeten, if desired), one tablespoon of granulated lecithin, and about five drops of lemon juice.

Blend all ingredients well. The granulated lecithin serves as an emulsifier and taste-improver. If you are allergic to soy, you can also use one tablespoon of raw-food quality almond powder. Can also be served as a dip for carrot or celery sticks.

Variation: If you like, you can also refine this sauce with garlic, grated horseradish, or dill.

Top Salad Dressing

This delicious salad dressing requires four tablespoons of cereal flakes, six tablespoons of cold-pressed olive oil, one pinch of herb salt, one pinch of freshly ground pepper or "papaya pepper" from dried papaya seeds, one pinch of freshly ground thyme, two garlic cloves that have been finely chopped and put through the garlic press, three tablespoons of barley grass juice, and, if desired, the juice of half a lemon.

First stir the flakes into the olive oil until it is smooth. Then add the salt, pepper, thyme, and garlic to it. Use a whisk to mix in the barley grass juice and lemon juice. This sauce can be kept for up to two days in the refrigerator.

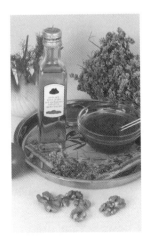

Vinaigrette Sauce with Barley Grass Juice

Take two tablespoons of apple cider vinegar or lemon juice and four tablespoons of cold-pressed oil, fresh herbs like chives, parsley, dill, chervil, or barley grass. Add two tablespoons of barley grass juice, two small shallots, some salt, and one pinch of pepper or "papaya pepper". If desired, add one grated garlic clove.

Finely chop herbs and mix with other ingredients.

Chocolate-Barley Grass Brittle
(Recipe from Halima Neumann)

Take three tablespoons of barley grass powder, two tablespoons of almond-milk powder, one tablespoon of carob powder (organic quality), and three tablespoons of high-quality olive oil or hemp oil (natural foods store). Mix almond-milk powder well with carob and oil to make smooth mixture, then add one tablespoon granulated lecithin or 1/2 avocado to strengthen the nerves. This nutritious dip is ideal food for the bones and brain. It can be used with apples and berries that are not too sweet or raw vegetables and salads.

Solid Foods

Young, tender barley grass blades (dried gently) can be chopped small and eaten like chives on whole-grain bread. Instead of butter, use mashed avocado as a spread. Moisten and chew well! Soups (cooled to body temperature), sauces, and salads can also have their health benefits improved by adding barley grass or wheat grass sprouts.

Barley Sprout-Barley Grass Power Breakfast

Use 1/2 of a cubed papaya, 1/2 of a chopped mango, one slice of fresh pineapple cut into cubes, 100 g of barley sprouts, one tablespoon of young, finely cut barley grass or one tablespoon of barley grass powder, one tablespoon of sprouted sunflower seeds, two tablespoons of cream (organic quality) or sweet-almond powder of a raw-food quality.

Mix the fruit with the barley grass, the barley juice, the barley sprouts, and the sunflower seeds. Possibly flavor with vanilla powder. Contains much vitamin E, vitamin C, and other vitamins, as well as many enzymes. Satisfies for hours.

Essene Flat Bread

Use approx. 700 g of two-day old barley or wheat sprouts, up to 800 g of kombucha drink or water, three teaspoons of nori algae, one tablespoon of barley grass powder, and coriander, garlic, and herbs of the season, according to taste.

Grind the sprouts in the mixer or a grain mill (made of metal) and knead in the barley grass powder, kombucha drink, algae, and spices by hand. Spread a 1/2-inch layer of this mixture onto a lightly oiled baking tin or in the fruit-drying machine (place wax paper beneath it). Cut into 2-inch squares before drying, then let dry at 40 degrees C for 14 to 16 hours. If you would like to dry the flat bread in the oven, select the lowest temperature and stick a wooden spoon in the door for better ventilation.

Chickpea Bread, Raw-Food Quality

Use 400 g of chick-pea sprouts, 400 g of wheat sprouts, 800 g of kombucha drink or water, one teaspoon of cumin, one pressed garlic clove, and one tablespoon of barley grass powder. For preparation, see "Essene Flat Bread."

Green Almond Cream
(Recipe from Halima Neumann)

Use two tablespoons of barley grass powder for this recipe. Add one tablespoon of almond milk powder, three tablespoons of pumpkin-seed or mild olive oil, and about 50 g of freshly chopped lemon balm or mint. Stir all ingredients together until creamy. This cream is excellent food for the nerves and a relaxant. It tastes delicious with raw fennel or celery sticks or steamed vegetables.

Chocolate-Pumpkin Barley Grass Cubes
(Recipe from Halima Neumann)

This recipe requires two tablespoons of barley grass powder, one tablespoon of almond milk powder, one tablespoon of carob powder, three tablespoons of sugar-free applesauce, three tablespoons of pumpkinseed oil, and two cups of cubed pumpkin (or turnip). Mix all other ingredients until creamy, then add the peeled pumpkin pieces. Sprinkle two tablespoons of cereal flakes on top. This goes well with pieces of apple (sour types) or raw vegetables or steamed vegetables such as fennel, fresh sweet corn, carrots, red beets, or parsley root. Strengthens bladder and kidneys, as well as eyes.

Herb Paste
(Recipe from Halima Neumann)

Use three tablespoons of hemp oil or four tablespoons of olive oil, four tablespoons of red-beet and celery juice or tomato juice from unheated tomatoes, three to four tablespoons of barley grass powder, and finely chopped onions or grated horseradish. If desired, ginger, lemon juice, and one pinch of sea salt. Stir everything until creamy and season with finely minced mint, basil, coriander herb, or chives. This is a delicious dip for any type of vegetable, salads, sprout salads, or even use as a taste spread for bread. This herb paste contains all of the amino acids.

Barley Grass Delight
(Recipe from Halima Neumann)

Take one ripe papaya, one to two grated apples or sugar-free applesauce, some ginger (fresh or 1/2 teaspoon of powder), and two tablespoons of barley grass powder. Mix papaya pieces with the apple and ginger, then stir in barley grass powder.

For lymph cleansing, eat one to two grapefruits or fresh pineapple (not too sweet) along with it and chew 20 to 30 black papaya seeds (or one teaspoon of papaya-seed powder).

Barley Grass Gazpacho
(Recipe from Halima Neumann)

For this recipe, use two to three peeled tomatoes, one ripe avocado, 200 g of grated cucumber or zucchini, about 50 g of finely minced onion, and three to four tablespoons of barley grass powder. Mash tomatoes together with avocado, cucumber, and add onion. Mix in barley grass powder. If desired, season with a pinch of salt or cress. Delicious with all types of vegetables and salads, pulses, legumes, and sprouts.

Mild Barley Grass Salad

This recipe requires three cups of freshly chopped barley grass, one finely chopped broccoli rose, two cubed tomatoes, one finely chopped bell pepper, one grated salad onion, and one cup of unseasoned steamed or sprouted natural rice.

Mix the salad ingredients thoroughly in a bowl. Add the Top Salad Dressing (see above) with the barley grass juice, and let everything soak for 10 minutes. This salad is very good for people with high blood pressure or blood pressure fluctuations. It also contains much vitamin E and provitamin A, as well as an abundance of minerals and enzymes. Salads like this are offered in spa clinics and sanatoriums in the USA. They are also popular with top athletes.

"Verona" Salad Plate

Use sweet corn kernels, grated carrot, finely chopped broccoli rosettes, cubed red bell pepper, one tablespoon of barley grass, four tablespoons of barley or wheat sprouts, and two tablespoons of pot herbs or wild herbs.

Mix the corn, carrots, broccoli, and bell pepper. Sprinkle with finely chopped barley grass, sprouts, and herbs.

Stuffed Bell Peppers

This recipe requires one large bell pepper per person. Cut off the "hats" and fill with the other ingredients.

In addition to the four bell peppers, the other ingredients are one finely chopped onion, 200 g finely chopped mushrooms, 200 g finely chopped cucumbers, some pepper, three tablespoons of finely chopped barley grass, one bunch of finely chopped chervil, two tablespoons of finely chopped fresh sage, two tablespoons of sunflower-seed or pumpkin-seed oil, 200 g of barley sprouts or wheat sprouts, and one squirt of tamari (soy sauce).

Mix all ingredients well in a bowl and stuff mixture into the bell peppers. If desired, serve with natural rice that has been steamed on a low flame.

BARLEY GRASS FROM A TO Z

This section does not claim to be complete. After decades of observing its effect, Dr. Yoshihide Hagiwara discovered that barley grass juice can improve or heal literally hundreds of different complaints and health problems. This even includes health disorders that hadn't responded to conventional therapy. Barley grass has such an extensive range of indications that it comprehensively strengthens and fortifies the powers of self-healing and the body's immune system from the inside out; it also activates and harmonizes all of the body's own regulating mechanisms. This is why taking barley grass should be seen, above all, from the perspective of preventive health care. Dr. Yoshihide Hagiwara writes that preventive medicine, which improves the constitution of the body, is more important today than any past period in the history of humanity.

In order to become truly healthy and remain truly healthy, we should not just depend upon synthetic pharmaceutics or isolated vitamin tablets, which can often have health-damaging side effects. It is apparent that the positive effects of raw green on our health cannot be replaced by any other type of food. At the same time, raw greens are completely free of side effects—except for the "side effect" of radiant health!

Instead of relying upon substances from the chemical laboratories, we should develop a natural protection against disease with the potent barley grass juice, for example. We can succeed in developing this by keeping our body healthy with a natural diet rich in vital substances.

In the USA, natural food stores have entire departments full of natural food supplements, the most predominant of which are green food supplements. As complete, holistic food supplements, "super food supplements" such as barley grass, wheat grass, blue-green algae, chlorella, and kamut fill the nutritional gaps created by our hectic lifestyle. They are rapidly becoming part of the American—and the international—diet.

Acidosis (Hyperacidity)

Barley grass is one of the most alkaline, if not *the* most alkaline, foods that exists. Alkaline-rich green juices alkalize the entire organism and neutralize acids. This also makes us more emotionally balanced and we don't have such an "acidic" response (also see chapter in this book "Restoring the Acid-Alcaline Balance with Barley Grass Juice" on page 96 ff.). Hyperacidity causes the tissue and the organs to "wilt," but the alkaline barley grass juice is like warm rain on a piece of dry land: a long-term rejuvenation of the skin and hair takes place from the inside out.

Alcoholism

In the long run, alcoholism destroys the liver. Grass juices are rich in mineral salts and chlorophyll, which are capable of regenerating the liver and repairing some of the damage that has been done. In addition, former alcoholics attain a renewed courage to face life and improved memory.

Anemia *see "Blood Cells, Formation of"*

Animals

Pets can also profit from barley grass. If they like it, they can either be given barley grass tablets or have the barley grass powder mixed into their feed or drinking water. This binds bad smells, which plague older dogs in particular. The digestive enhancers in most barley grass powder maintain well-regulated digestion. The many minerals in barley grass juice balance the excess acids of canned food on a meat basis. Most cat food and dog food contains too little dietary fiber. With barley grass, cat and dog fur will become shiny again. The eyes become radiant and the animals develop more joy and vitality.

One pleasant accompanying effect: cats stop chewing on houseplants. When I take care of dogs and cats, I put a tray of fresh, homegrown barley grass outside so they can help themselves to it. Or, I reserve part of the garden in summer for them by planting a special plot of barley grass. I give my children's pygmy rabbits one small tablet of barley grass each every other day, which they greedily nibble away. Green Magma is available for dogs and cats as the products, Barley Cat and Barley Dog. I have successfully tested these products on our two cats and on my friends' animals. The rate of acceptance and the effect on the pets are excellent.

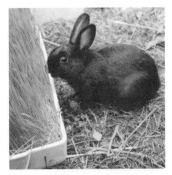

Wounds can also be healed by placing a ground or chewed bunch of barley grass (alternative: a cotton-

The little rabbits like to snack on the author's homegrown barley grass

wool pad soaked with barley grass juice) on the wound and holding it in place with a bandage. The bandage should be renewed every two to three hours. If an animal has skin problems, dab the area with a cotton-wool pad that has been soaked in barley grass juice and slightly wrung out. This helps against such ailments as eczema, for example.

There have been reports of horses cured of their blindness by letting them graze in a meadow with young cereal grasses.

Athletes

In the USA, barley grass is considered the ideal food and medicine for athletes. Leisure-time athletes can also profit from this knowledge because every athletic activity increases the formation of free radicals, which can be held in check by the antioxidants contained in barley grass. Especially the enzymes SOD, catalase, and glutathione peroxidase, all of which are contained in barley grass, prevent cell membrane in the muscles from becoming damaged by free-radicals. Taking barley grass also prevents inflammations and enables the body to achieve its top performance.[66]

Many athletes are switching from sugared, electrolytic sport drinks to barley grass juice. It gives them more energy that is slowly released in the body, and they experience fatigue and exhaustion much less frequently. Many top athletes take barley grass on a regular basis: one example is Eric Baker of Boulder, Colorado, who won first place at the Iron Man in New Zealand and at the Powerman in Zofingen, Switzerland in 1994. Other famous U.S. athletes who drink barley grass juice on a regular basis are David Hawk (bodybuilder) and Jerry Dunn (marathon runner). Also see "Sports."

Bad Breath

Barley grass juice binds bad breath and deodorizes it. The juice contains enzymes that have an antibacterial effect and chlorophyll binds smells. A barley grass therapy would also be good since bad breath usually comes from undigested food in the stomach. Barley grass tablets have proved useful when given to older dogs, which frequently develop an intolerable smell from their mouths. Barley grass powder can also be mixed into pet food. They will be more likely to accept this with Green Magma.

Blood Cells, Formation of

Chlorophyll, which is abundant in barley grass, has a blood-cell forming effect within the body. Chlorophyll as an isolated substance and iron preparations are ineffective because copper, which is amply available in barley grass, is required to store iron in the hemoglobin. When there is a copper or iron deficiency, anemia develops. Many women in particular suffer from this health disorder. The copper from barley grass and other dark-green plants is also important for the color pigmentation in the skin and hair. Dr. Ann Wigmore, who had gray hair at an early age, returned to her original hair color through green plant foods when she was over 60 years of age!

Brain

Chlorophyll-containing food such as barley grass enriches the blood with oxygen and thereby helping to enhance brain function. The amino acid, glutamic acid, especially abundant in barley grass, plays a wide range of roles in brain activity. In addition to its critical role in energy production in the brain, glutamic acid acts as an excitatory neurotransmitter mediating motor activity and memory storage and retrieval processes. It is also successfully used as turbo-fuel for the brain in cases of concentration disorders, senility, depression, states of exhaustion, and impotence. At the same time, glutamic acid reduces the desire for harmful substances like alcohol, nicotine, sweets, and drugs.

Another amino acid contained in barley grass, phenylalanine, is recommended and used by orthomolecular medicine as a remedy for improving the memory, reducing feelings of hunger, and against depression. Phenylalanine's actions in facilitating brain activity may be due to its conversion to tyrosine, a precursor for the synthesis of the neurotransmitter, norepinephrine. Barley grass provides additional important brain food such as magnesium, potassium, sodium, vitamin C, and zinc.

Children

Green foods like barley grass are especially important for children. Barley grass juice has the same pH value as breast milk. My son Michael, who is 13 years old, always takes barley grass tablets to school with him. The amino-acid that they contain, such as glutamic acid, stimulates the brain functions. Many hyperactive and unruly children probably suffer from hyperacidity. Barley grass juice helps restore their acid-alkaline balance and lets them become relaxed, peaceful, and cheerful. Halima Neumann believes that a disturbed brain metabolism is responsible for the development of neurosis: "save your children's minds!" The exorphin content (exorphins are morphine-like addictive substances)—such as that in cow's milk, meat, and wheat—apparently leads to abnormal functional processes in the brain with the resulting behavioral disorders. Delicious recipes with alternative foods such as almond milk can be found in the recipe section of this book, on page 116 ff.

Cleansing *see Removal of Waste Substances*

Diabetes

People with diabetes have had good experiences using barley grass. Taking it on a regular basis normalizes the blood-sugar level. Similar good results can also be achieved with blue-green algae powder. For both of these foods, normalization of the blood-sugar level is attributed to the quickly available nutrients of mucopolysaccharides and especially the effect of the trace elements manganese and zinc (important for insulin storage, wound-healing, and strengthening of the immune system), as well as chromium (important for carbohydrate metabolism). The attempt to improve glucose tolerance with synthetically produced chromium compounds has failed. In order to have the proper effect, chromium must be absorbed in the form of the so-called glucose tolerance factor (GTF), which is abundantly available in barley grass, stevia, and blue-green algae.

The high proportion of enzyme complexes in barley grass and blue-green algae stimulate the activity of the pancreas. Ripe papaya or unripe green papaya, grated as apple-papaya herb, have an especially healing and strengthening effect for the exhausted pancreas; they can stimulate the endogenous (body's own) production of enzymes in a natural manner. All chemically processed foods, alcohol, salt, and medications rob the body of its enzymes. Other enzyme-robbers are cooked foods since the enzymes are destroyed by heat. Enzyme-rich raw plant foods such as barley grass juice, nut proteins, and raw fruit support the healing process for diabetes.

A deficiency of all the B vitamins, vitamin C, and vitamin A, as well as a lack of manganese, has been discovered in diabetics. All of these vitamins, as well as selenium, are amply present in barley grass juice. Instead of margarine with its harmful trans-fatty acids, diabetics should use avocado as a bread spread. (Together with easily digested fat, avocado also contains abundant lecithin as food for the nerves and brain, as well as vitamin E.) In addition to vitamin C and selenium, vitamin E is an especially potent scavenger of cell-destroying free radicals. According to Halima Neumann, almost all diabetics have a candida fungal overgrowth in their intestines. Consequently, diabetics should not drink wheat grass juice.

Digestive Problems

The enzymes in barley grass juice stimulate exhausted digestive glands in a natural way and optimize the manner in which food is utilized. When the barley grass powder contains dietary fiber (see product information), digestion is additionally stimulated and constipation is no longer a problem. Through its balanced portions of potassium and sodium, barley grass activates peristalsis (wavelike muscular contractions of the intestine): potassium causes expansion and sodium causes contractions.

Furthermore, the chlorophyll in barley grass binds unpleasant smells in the case of flatulence since it has a deodorizing effect. Barley grass juice promotes the body's own formation of vitamin B12 and regeneration of the intestinal flora. This is because of the way chlorophyll helps resettle the intestines with aerobic, oxygen-loving bacteria that are vital for controlling the anaerobic bacteria and parasites like candida, cancer cells and viruses.

Drug Addiction

Dr. Ann Wigmore had particularly good experiences with wheat grass and barley grass for drug addicts, including many young people. The high proportion of calcium, magnesium, phosphorus, and potassium apparently helps to eliminate drug residue from the organs, muscle tissue, and connective tissue. Through the abundance of supplied minerals, the body restores its acid-alkaline balance and the human being become more psychologically balanced and stable. This gives him or her greater chances of getting away from all types of drugs. On the Internet, there are many personal stories of how consumers of barley grass juice were able to give up smoking, for example, within a short period of time.[67]

Fasting

Fasting can be a pleasure with barley grass. Since barley grass contains an abundance of minerals, vitamins, and proteins, we can continue to provide the body with vital substances while it cleanses itself and the intestines are given a rest. The feared healing crises such as headache or dizziness do not occur or are considerably eased. As needed, drink barley grass juice, either from fresh barley leaves or powder mixed with water, three to four times a day. Green Magma is especially well suited for this purpose because it does not contain the dietary fiber. More information about barley grass fasting can be found in the chapter "Recipes with Barley Grass" on page 116 ff.

Fatigue, Exhaustion

When they are tired, many people eat sweets or push themselves by drinking beverages containing caffeine. They set the "sugar swing" in motion and within a short time, they feel even more tired than before. Chlorophyll-containing grass juices are a healthy alternative. They contain an abundance of vitamins, minerals, and enzymes that are the ideal brain food. They also activate the liver, which provides the body with energy (also see Brain).

Chronic fatigue is not normal and usually is a result of an unhealthy diet and lifestyle. With the help of barley grass juice, you can attain a high energy level within two days because the grass juice balances the nutritionally-caused deficiency symptoms and removes waste substances that may be harming the body's cells, blood, tissue, and organs. If we supplement our diet with barley grass and raw fruits and vegetables, our cells store a maximum electrical charge and we have plenty of energy available to us. Through light and foods that are alive, such as barley grass juice, which optimally nourish and cleanse our body, the need for sleep is reduced to six hours or less; we feel full of energy and joy when we awake.

Other very effective methods for increasing the joy in life are the authentic Reiki® and the yoga rituals in the Five Tibetan Rites.

Gums, Inflammation of the (Gingivitis)

Gargle barley grass juice or very slowly chew the juice out of a bunch of barley grass to counteract inflammation of the gums. The enzymes contained in the juice have an anti-inflammatory and anti-bacterial effect.

Hyperacidity

Barley grass juice is one of the most effective natural remedies for successfully encountering the widespread disease of hyperacidity. Chemical remedies against heartburn, which are purchased for millions of dollars annually, are not therapy for the cause of the problem since they neutralize the digestive juices for hours. In addition, stomach remedies with the active ingredient of Cisaprid can have serious side-effects: If the afflicted party also swallows antibiotics, life-threatening fibrillation of the heart chamber may even occur. Furthermore, acidic gastric acid is necessary for the digestion of proteins. Neutralizing the gastric acid with medication has the following result: the chyme remains in the stomach too long and begins to ferment. The fermentation acid attacks the mucous membranes, which are already damaged, and can lead to gastritis in the worst case. Another negative consequence is the recurring toxification through the intestines into the blood because of protein putrefaction in the small and large intestine.

This evil can be attacked at the root with green barley grass juice since all of the glandular functions are dependent upon the proper pH value and barley grass restores the optimal acid-alkaline balance. (Also see Acidosis.)

Immune System

The chlorophyll and the vitamin- and enzyme-complex in barley grass uniquely strengthen our defensive system. The enzyme complexes in barley green have an antioxidant effect, meaning that they successfully fight cell-deteriorating oxygen compounds, the free radicals. Beta carotene, which is richly present in barley grass, stimulates the bacteria-fighter lysozyme and the production of T-lymphocytes; vitamin B1 is important for the functioning of the lymph system with its detoxification function; vitamin B2 (riboflavin), amply present in barley grass, stimulates the activities of the antibodies; vitamin B6 (pyridoxine) strengthens our immune system; folic acid is important for fighting cancer cells and for the production of defensive cells; choline, also abundantly available in barley grass, strengthens the hormone production and its defensive strength; vitamin C helps the phagocytes get to where they are needed and promotes the effectiveness of the killer cells; copper strengthens our immune system; so does iron, which provides the defensive cells with the necessary oxygen; zinc, also amply present in barley grass, primarily stimulates the defensive power of the T cells, which are produced in the thymus gland.

When people have cancer or AIDS, their bodies require many of the easily assimilable short chained of amino acids, which are called polypeptides. The body mainly uses these in order to create defensive cells (T lymphocytes). Barley grass is also enrichment for the weakened immune systems when people suffer from allergies or diabetes. The biological availability of the polypeptides in barley grass, as well as that in blue-green algae and kamut/halmit green (primal wheat grass) is unsurpassed.

Infections

Chlorophyll is the ideal food for preventing and healing all types of infections. The immune system is activated and stimulated by the abundance of vitamin C and beta carotene in grass juices.

Intestines

Barley grass juice is a blessing for the intestines. It cleanses the intestines of protein residue and other waste substances with its high proportion of chlorophyll, ensuring that the healthy intestinal flora can flourish. Cereal grasses like barley grass are used in laboratories throughout the world as remedies for promoting the growth of lactobacilli, the desired healthy intestinal bacteria. Barley grass also helps to restore intestinal flora that has been damaged by penicillin and to stop the growth of harmful bacteria and fungi in the intestines. Through the high proportion of roughage in most barley grass juice products, the intestinal passage is accelerated. This prevents intestinal cancer and constipation (also see "Digestion"). Barley grass powder is one of the few digestive enhancers rich food supplements that provide a balanced mixture of vitamins, minerals, and proteins in addition to dietary fiber.

Libido *see Sexuality*

Malnutrition and Poor Nutrition

Many people in the industrial nations are "starving in front of full pots." They eat too many "empty" calories, fat, and animal protein, along with too little of the vital substances, which are primarily found in fruits and vegetables. Through the lack of vitamins and minerals in our food (for example: the vitamin-C content of apples sank by 80% during recent years; see chapter on vitamins on page 76 ff.), deficiencies in vital substances are preprogrammed. Because of the increasingly negative living conditions with much smog, noise, and stress, we need considerably *more* vitamins, minerals, and other vital substances than ever before. In order to prevent disease and the symptoms of premature aging, it is best to give the body a diet of much fresh fruit and vegetables together with a high-dosage, natural, and balanced food supplement like barley grass juice.

There have been very positive experiences using wheat grass or barley grass juice for people who are undernourished; however, these juices should only be given to them in small amounts diluted with three parts water to one part juice in order to avoid excessively quick detoxification of the weakened eliminatory organs.

Osteoporosis

Barley grass provides calcium that is optimally available for effective prevention of osteoporosis. Regeneration of the tissue, skeleton, and cartilage is dependent upon a balanced relationship between vitamin C, proteins, and magnesium. Although sheep, horse, and goat's milk that has not been heated represents a good source of calcium and magnesium, it does not provide the necessary vitamin C. The use of dairy products for osteoporosis prevention must be strongly discouraged since cow's milk does not contain magnesium and its calcium has become inorganic through heating (pasteurization, homogenization, boiling). This can lead to calcium deposits, sometimes called "milk gout," and kidney stones.

Moreover, milk contains too much phosphorus in relation to calcium and the excess phosphates combine with the calcium into insoluble salts that are eliminated at best; otherwise, they are deposited in the body as waste substances.

In addition to barley grass, blue-green algae powder, alfalfa sprouts, sesame, peeled almonds, avocado, nettle seeds, bananas, and comfrey are excellent plant sources of calcium.

Overweight *see Weight Problems*

Rejuvenation: Slowing Down the Aging Process

The cell-protecting enzymes in barley grass render the cell-attacking free radicals harmless and accelerate the process of cell renewal. A special role is played in this process by the enzyme superoxide dismutase (SOD), which is amply present in barley grass. (Also see chapters on "Barley Grass Juice, a Rejuvenation Elixir" on page 100 ff. and "Superoxide Dismutase (SOD)—A Wonder Remedy? on page 94 ff. in this book.) Barley grass contains an especially high amount of polypeptides, short-chain amino acids that our body needs as building blocks for new cells.

Removal of Waste Substances, Detoxification

Barley grass juice especially promotes the detoxification of the liver, lymph, kidneys, and digestive organs. Barley grass supports better digestion and utilization of the food, increasing the speed at which catabolic products are eliminated.

Sexuality, Libido

Barley grass contains much zinc and therefore strengthens the production of seminal fluid and male sexual energy. Its content of isoflavonoids, which have an estrogen-like effect, benefits the formation of secondary female sex characters and the development of the milk-duct system of the breasts, as well as the libido in both men and women. Dr. Yoshihide Hagiwara observed that women with underdeveloped breasts achieved larger breasts by drinking barley grass juice. A tip for women: Serve your partner a drink of barley grass extract or freshly squeezed barley juice three times a day! You will probably never have to complain about boredom in the bedroom again. (Also see Sexual Potency.)

Dr. Yoshihide Hagiwara and Dr. Mary Ruth Swope report about men who have had their potency and libido restored after a few weeks of taking barley grass juice. And this occurred without any type of side-effects except for being more fit and energy-charged than before!

The isoflavonoids contained in barley grass juice stabilize fluctuations in the female hormonal balance. This makes barley grass juice an outstanding natural remedy for women to prevent menopausal complaints such as loss of libido, hot flashes, etc.

Sexual Potency

In animal experiments, Dr. Yoshihide Hagiwara discovered that when mice were given green barley essence they developed more healthy sperm than the control group. The function of the reproductive glands was apparently strengthened and stimulated since barley grass juice contains many isoflavonoids, an estrogen-like substance. Barley grass also contains the amino acid arginine, which is particularly important for men's fertility because large amounts of it are found in seminal fluid. Dr. Yoshihide Hagiwara also observed that the muscle functions of both women and men were strengthened, probably through the potassium in barley grass, which is also beneficial for the movements during sexual intercourse and the ability to have an orgasm. (Also see Sexuality.)

The animal-protection organization Peta recommends that men should switch to a vegetarian diet in order to maintain their potency up into ripe old age. According to Peta, meat leads to arteriosclerosis and this has the drastic consequence of impotence.

Skin

With its abundance of vitamins, minerals, enzymes, proteins, and chlorophyll, barley grass improves all of the body functions. It detoxifies the body, which manifests itself in skin that is more attractive, smoother, and has better circulation. The barley grass enzymes improve cutaneous respiration and renew the skin so that it looks younger. Wrinkles smooth out. To combat acne, skin impurities, skin inflammations, eczemas, and neurodermatitis, applying external cotton-wool compresses soaked in barley grass juice has proved to be a successful method. In Japan, there is already a cosmetic series based on barley grass juice. Cosmetic products on a papaya basis are also suitable for the above skin problems. See my book *Healing Power of Papaya* (Bibliography on page 147).

Sports *see Athletes*

Green juices from algae and cereal grasses have become "green manna," which provides quickly available energy without digestive strain, for both top athletes and leisure-time athletes in the USA. This energy burns slowly and enables them to achieve their best athletic performances. In addition, the polypeptides, easily digestible proteins present in barley grass, build up the muscles. Because of this, barley grass is considered a "natural anabolic agent" in the USA and Canada. The protein powders enriched with sugar or glucose that are available in fitness studios and sports sections of department stores only set the sugar swing in motion; as a result, they only deliver short-term energy. With their composition, they can never approach the synergistic action mechanism of plant proteins in raw-food quality.

In addition, barley grass juice replaces the large amounts of minerals that are lost through perspiration and prevents muscle cramps since it works against the hyperacidity (see Acidosis) created by muscle work.

I am in my late-forties and make myself a barley grass/blue-green algae beverage that I drink at least three times a day. I have no problems jogging over an hour at a time, even in mountainous areas.

Stress

Barley grass is an excellent remedy to help us react serenely in stressful situations. And who *doesn't* suffer from stress in our fast-paced and performance-oriented society?

Barley grass is a balanced food with a high concentration of nutrients. It stabilizes the body both physically and mentally, reducing the tendency toward overreactions and neuroses. Through the adrenaline output in stress situations, the body has an increased elimination of minerals and vitamins, especially B vitamins. Barley grass juice can replenish this deficit within a short amount of time. If we achieve an acid-alkali balance through daily consumption of barley grass juice (see the chapter on "Restoring the Acid-Alkaline Balance with Barley Grass Juice" in this book, on page 96 ff.), we also do not react as "acidly" in the psychological sense and remain calm and cheerful in stress situations.

In addition to taking barley grass, a good way to prevent stress is endurance training, such as jogging (best in the morning) on a regular basis and learning a simple, effective relaxation technique such as the authentic Reiki®. (I hold lectures and seminars about this method in the USA as well.)

Vegetarians

Vegetarians often suffer from a lack of vitamin B12, folic acid, iron, and potassium—especially "pudding vegetarians" who simply just leave out the meat and eat very little raw fruits and vegetables with their related vital substances. Barley grass juice, either fresh or as a ready-to-mix powder, makes it possible to balance nutrient deficiencies and provide ourselves with the necessary vital substances. Barley grass is one of the few plant sources containing vitamin B12, an important "nerve vitamin."

Weight Problems, Obesity

The fat-splitting enzymes in the body are activated by the enzyme complexes contained in barley grass juice. Furthermore, the portion of cholesterol-lowering gamma-linolenic acid and essential linoleic acid contributes to the reduction of excessive fat. The lipid metabolism is accelerated by barley grass juice, which makes it easier to control weight. Both of the amino acids glutaminic acid and phenylalanine curb feelings of hunger and are used in orthomolecular medicine for weight reduction. The chromium and zinc in barley grass, as well as the minerals magnesium and manganese, normalize the blood-sugar level.

The outstandingly strong nutrient profile of barley grass satisfies the appetite for hours. For weight-reducing purposes, two tablespoons of barley grass powder replace one complete meal. The barley grass powder can also be stirred into a red beet-celery juice mixture or mouth-temperature vegetable broth or miso soup. If you like it fruity, you can also chop up one-fourth of a pineapple with one sour apple (like a Boskop) and juice it in the blender. When traveling or at the office, you can stir the barley grass powder into sugar-free applesauce. One tablespoon of granulated soy-lecithin can also be added for increased reduction of fat. Instead of two tablespoons of barley grass powder, you can also use one tablespoon of blue-green algae powder and one tablespoon of barley grass powder.

Endurance training such as jogging is recommended for stimulating the metabolism. The authentic Reiki® can be practiced to harmonize the functioning of the thyroid gland.

APPENDIX

Bibliography

Magazine Articles

"Barley Is a Time-Honored Remedy for Athletes." In: *Better Nutrition*, November 1995.

Chichoke, Anthony: "Green Barley Extract: A Study in Quality." In: *Showcase Magazine*, without date.

Chichoke, Anthony: "The Green Genie in a Bottle." In: *Total Health*, vol. 16, No. 2, April 1994.

Chichoke, Anthony: "The Ideal Fast Food with an Antioxidant Twist." In: *Townsend Letter for Doctors*, July 1994.

"Enzymatic Green Salad in a Bottle—The Flu/Cold Fighter." In: *Let's Live*, October 1994.

Gornley, James J.: "Green Barley. Green Gold. Mining a Nutritional Motherlode." In: *Better Nutrition*, July 1996.

"Green Barley Grass May Help Arthritics." In: *Better Nutrition for Today's Living*, July 1995.

"Green Barley Is Rich in Enzymes, Nutrients for Improving Vitality." In: *Better Nutrition*, January 1996.

"Green Waves of Barley Ease Arthritis for Some." In: *Better Nutrition for Today's Living*, September 1995.

Scheer, James F.: "Green is Gold for a Healthful Diet." In: *Better Nutrition*, April 1995.

Seibold, Ronald L.: "There's More than One Way to Get Your Greens." In: *Better Nutrition*, September 1996.

Hartman, Stephen: "Barley Grass: Nature's Own Antacid." In: *Healthy & Natural Journal*.

"Wonderful Experience with Green Magma." Lectures by: Pejic, Lassen, Estrada and Weigel, YH Products Corporation, 1986.

Books

Balch, James F. and Balch, Phyllis A.: *Prescription for Nutritional Health*, Avery Publishing Group, New York, 1997.

Chopra, Deepak: *Perfect Health: The Complete Mind/Body Guide*, Harmony Books, New York, 1990.

Chopra, Deepak: *The Seven Spiritual Laws of Success*, Amber-Allen Publ., 1995

Clement, Brian R.: *Hippocrates Health Program—A Proven Guide to Healthful Living*, Hippocrates Publishing, West Palm Beach, 1992.

Cichoke, Anthony J.: *Enzymes & Enzyme Therapy*, Keats Publishing, New Canaan, 1994.

Cousens, Dr. Gabriel: *Spiritual Nutrition and the Rainbow Diet*, Cassandra Press, 1987.

Diamond, Harvey and Diamond Marilyn: *Fit for Life*, Warner Books, New York, 1985.

Eftekhar, Judy Lin: *Feed Yourself Right!*, Globe Communications Corp., Boca Raton, 1997.

Gerson, Dr. Max: *A Cancer Therapy: Results of 50 Cases and the Cure of Advanced Cancer*, Talman Co., 1997.

Hagiwara, Dr. Yoshihide: *Green Barley Essence—The Ideal 'Fast Food'*, Keats Publishing, New Canaan, 1985.

Heinerman, John: *Heinerman's Encyclopedia of Juices, Teas & Tonics*, Prentice Hall, Englewood Cliffs, 1996.

Heinerman, John: *Heinerman's Encyclopedia of Healing Juices*, Parker Publishing, West Nyack, 1994.

Howell, Dr. Edward: *Enzyme Nutrition—The Food Enzyme Concept*, Avery Publishing Group, Wayne, New Jersey, 1985.

Kulvinskas, Viktoras and Taska, Richard Jr.: *Survival into the 21st Century*, Twenty First Century Publ., ISBN 0933278047, 1975.

Malkmus, Dr. Gerorge H: *Why Christians Get Sick*, Treasure House, Shippensburg, 6th edition, 1997.

Markowitz, Elysa: *Living with Green Power. A Gourmet Collection of Living Food Recipes*, Alive Books, Canada, 1997.

Meyerowitz, Steve: *Wheat Grass, Nature's First Medicine. The Complete Guide to Using Grasses to Revitalize Your Health*, Sproutman Publications, Great Barrington, Massachusetts, 1998.

Mother Meera: *Answers*, Part I, Meeramma Publ., ISBN 0962297733X.

Murray, Frank: *Hagiwara, Yoshihide—Pioneer of Better Living*, Keats Publishing, New Canaan, 1990.

Neumann, Halima: *Stop Krebs, MS, Aids, Eine neue Ganzheitsmethode*, Fürhoff-Verlag, Starnberg, 1997.

Neumann, Halima: *Stop der Azidose, Allergien und Haarausfall*, Fürhoff, Starnberg, 4th edition, 1994.

Neumann, Halima: *Grüne Lebensenergien—Heilkraft aus dem Schoß der Erde*, Führhoff, Starnberg, 1999.

Ray, Dr. Barbara: *The Authentic Reiki*, Radiance Associates, St. Petersburg, 1997.

Seibold, Ronald L.: *Cereal Grass—What's in It for You!*, Wilderness Community Education Foundation, Lawrence, 1990.

Sharamon, Shalila and Baginski, Bodo J.: *The Healing Power of Grapefruit Seed*, Lotus Light, Twin Lakes, WI, 1996.

Simonsohn, Barbara: *Healing Power of Papaya*, Lotus Press, Twin Lakes, WI, 2000.

Swope, Dr. Mary Ruth: *Green Leaves of Barley*, Dr. Swope Enterprises, Phoenix, 1990.

Swope, Dr. Mary Ruth: *The Spiritual Roots of Barley*, National Preventive Health Services, Melbourne, 1988.

Tietze, Harald W.: *Supreme Green Medicine*, Bermagui, 1998.

Ulmer, G.A.: *Gesundheitswunder Chlorophyll – Gespeicherte, gesundheitsspendende Sonnen- und Heilkraft*, Ulmer Verlag, Tuningen, Germany, 1997.

Walsch, Neale Donald: *Conversations with God—An Uncommon Dialogue*, Harper, San Francisco, 1994.

Wigmore, Ann: *The Wheatgrass Book*, Hippocrates Health Institute, 1985.

Wigmore, Ann: *The Hippocrates Diet and Health Program*, Avery Publishing Group, Wayne, 1984.

Wigmore, Ann: *Be Your Own Doctor*, Avery Publishing Group, Wayne, 1982.

Wigmore, Ann: *Why Suffer—How I Overcame Illness & Pain Naturally*, Avery Publishing Group, Wayne, 1985.

Research

Goldstein, Shibamoto, and Kubota, *Published Research Findings on Barley Leaf Extract*, Green Food Corporation, 1998.

Goldstein, Allan L.: *A Natural Food Supplement to Improve One's Health*, Nature's Laboratory, 1997.

Hagiwara, Dr. Yoshihide: *Study on Green Juice Powder of Young Barley Leaves II*, 98th Annual Assembly of Pharmaceutical Society of Japan, 1978.

Hagiwara, Dr. Yoshihide: *Prevention of Aging and Adult Diseases Methods for Longevity and Good Health*, The International Foundation for Preventive Medicine, New York, 1981.

Hagiwara, Dr. Yoshihide, Goldstein, Bao, Sprangelo und Badamchian: "Isolation of a Vitamin E Analog from a Green Barley Leaf Extract that Stimulates Release of Prolactin and Growth Hormone from Rat Anterior Pituitary Cells in Vitro." In: *Journal of Nutrition Biochemistry*, 1994.

Kitta, Dr. Hagiwara and Shibamoto: "Antioxidative Activity of an Isoflavonoid 2"-O-Glycosylisovitexin Isolated from Green Barley Leaves." In: *Journal of Agricultural and Food Chemistry*, Department of Environmental Toxicology, University of California, California, 1992.

Kubota, Kazuhiko and Matsuoka, Yutaka: *Effect of Chronic Administration of Green Barley Juice on Growth Rate, Serum Cholesterol Level and Internal Organs of Mice*, Science University of Tokyo, Japan.

Kubota, Kazuhiko and Matsuoka, Yutaka: *Isolation of Potent Anti-inflammatory Protein from Barley Leaves*, Science University of Tokyo, Japan, 1983.

Kubota and Sunagane: *Studies on the Effects of Green Barley Juice on the Endurance and Motor Activity in Mice*, Science University of Tokyo, Japan, 1984.

Kubota, Matsuoka and Seki: *Isolation of Potent Anti-inflammatory Protein from Barley Leaves*, Science University of Tokyo, Japan, 1983.

Muto, Tatsuo: *Therapeutic Experiment of Bakuryokuso for the Treatment of Skin Diseases in the Main,* New Drugs and Clinical Application, Tokyo, 1977.

Nishiyama, Tadashi: *Study of Young Barley Leaf Extract: The Antioxidative Compound and Its Effect*, Department of Environmental Toxicology, University of California, Davis, California, USA, July '91-June '93.

Nishiyama, Dr. Hagiwara and Shibamoto*: Inhibition of Malonaldehyde Formation from Lipids by an Isoflavonoid Isolated from Young Green Barley Leaves,* Department of Environmental Toxicology, University of California, 1993.

Osawa, Katauzaki, Dr. Hagiwara, and Shibamoto: *A Novel Antioxidant Isolated from Young Green Barley Leaves*, Agricultural an Food Chemistry, 1992.

Ohtake, Yuasa, Komura, Miyauchi, Dr. Hagiwara and Kubota: *Studies on the Constituents of Green Juice from Young Barley Leaves*, Science University of Tokyo, Japan.

Ohtake, Nonaka, Sawada, Dr. Hagiwara and Kubota: *Studies on the Constituents of Green Juice from Young Barley Leaves—Effect on Dietarily Induces Hypercholesterolemia in Rats*, Science University of Tokyo, Japan.

Ohtake, Yuasa, Komura, Dr. Hagiwara and Kubota: *Studies on the Constituents of Green Juice from Young Barley Leaves—Antiulcer Activity of Fractions from Barley Juice*, Science University of Tokyo, Japan.

Shibamoto, Dr. Hagiwara und Osawa: *A Flavonoid with Strong Antioxidative Activity Isolated from Young Green Barley Leaves*, Department of Environmental Toxicology, University of California, California, 1994.

Yokono, Osamu: *Therapeutic Effect of Water-Soluble Form of Chlorophyll-A and the Related Substance. The Young Barley Green Juice in the Treatment of Patients with Chronic Pancreatitis*", Faculty of Medicine, University of Tokyo, Japan.

Notes

1. "Von wegen ein Apfel täglich!" in: *BIO*, 4/98, page 6.
2. Dr. Yoshihide Hagiwara: *Green Barley Essence—The Ideal Fast Food*.
3. Viktoras Kulvinskas: *Survival into the 21ˢᵗ Century*.
4. Ronald L. Seibold: *Cereal Grass—What's in It for You!*
5. See note 3.
6. See note 4
7. Ibid.
8. See note 2
9. Ibid.
10. H.G. Berner: *An vollen Töpfen verhungern*, page 21.
11. Ibid., page 20
12. Addresses: Living-Food Institute Skeppsgården, 61592 Valdenmarsvik, Sweden (classes in Swedish and English); Hyppocrates Health Institute, 1441 Palmdale Court, West Palm Beach, Florida 33411, phone: 407-471-8876, Ann Wigmore Foundation, 196 Commonwealth Avenue, Boston, MA 02116, phone: 617-267-9424, Dr. Ann Wigmore's Institute P.O. Box, 429, Puerto Rico 00677.
13. Halima Neumann: *Stop Krebs, MS, AIDS*.
14. Dr. Mary Ruth Swope: *Green Leaves of Barley*.
15. Dr. Tatsuo Muto's research *Therapeutic Experiment of Bakuryosuso (the young green barley juice). For Treatment of Skin Diseases in Man* was published in 1977.
16. See note 14, pages 125-127.
17. Mary Ruth Swope: *The Spiritual Roots of Barley*.
18. Ibid, page 42.
19. Ibid, page 115.
20. Dr. Gabriel Cousens: *Spiritual Nutrition and the Rainbow Diet*.
21. North Dakota Barley Council: *Barley, an Ancient Grain for Today's Lifestyle*, 1993 and *Barley, The World's Oldest Grain*, 1992.
22. See note 4.
23. James J. Gornley: *Green Barley. Green Gold. Mining a Nutritional Motherlode*.
24. See note 4.
25. Ibid.
26. Klaus P. Waldmann: *Natürlich heilen und gesund bleiben mit Weizengras*, page 8.
27. See note 4.
28. See note 2.
29. John Heinermann: *Encyclopedia of Healing Juices*, page 270.
30. *The Importance of Wheat Grass, Barley Grass and Other Green Vegetables in the Human Diet*, Wilderness Community Education Foundation, Inc., Lawrance, USA, 1990, page 16.
31. Ibid, page 272.
32. Contact addresses for both institutes: Daido Bldg., Room no. 303, 3-5-5, Uchikanda, Chiyoda-ku, Tokyo, 101, Japan, phone: 03256-8106.
33. See note 3.
34. See note 2.
35. Halima Neumann: *Grüne Lebensenergien—Heilkraft aus dem Schoß der Erde*, page 99.

36. Barbara Simonsohn: *Healing Power of Papaya.*

37. See note 14.

38. Dr. Edward Howell: *Enzyme Nutrition.*

39. See note 2.

40. See note 1.

41 See books of Dr. Mary Ruth Swope, Dr. Yoshihide Hagiwara and Halima Neuman.

42 Dr. Ann Wigmore: *The Wheatgrass Book.*

44 See note 4.

45 See note 2.

46 See the chapter in this book "Acidic Is Not Funny" on page 99 and the chapter on acidosis in my book *Healing Power of Papaya.*

47 See note 10, page 51.

48 See note 4.

49 G.A. Ulmer: *Gesundheitswunder Chlorophyll,* page 55.

50 See note 4.

51 See note 3.

52 Ibid.

53 See note 2 and note 14.

54 See note 2.

55 Ibid.

56 Halima Neumann: *Stop Krebs, MS, AIDS,* page 90.

57 Halima Heumann: *Stop der Azidose,* page 79.

58 See note 2 and 14.

59 See note 3.

60 Hans Kugler: *Slowing down the Aging Proc*ess.

61 See note 35.

62 See note 57, page 136.

63 See note 4.

64 See note 2.

65 Mother Meera: *Answers,* part I.

66 See article: "Barley Is a Time-Honored Remedy for Athlets" in: *Better Nutrition,* November 1995, page 170.

67 See http:wheatgrass.com/introtowg/testimonials.html

The Author

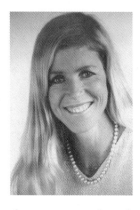

Barbara Simonsohn was born in January of 1954 as an Aquarius with a Sagittarius Ascendant. After completing high school, she studied sociology and concluded her studies as a political scientist.

She worked as a public relations manager for a large German organization that sponsors exchange programs for young people (Youth for Understanding) before she decided to learn about organic farming and gardening. For ten consecutive years, she spent several weeks at a time at the Findhorn Community in Scotland. Here she worked in the garden, attended seminars, and learned many holistic methods of healing such as Authentic Reiki.

For one-and-a-half years, she studied at the biodynamic organic farm of Baldur Springmann, one of the best-known organic farmers in Germany. Since the mid-Seventies, she has also written articles on these topics for German magazines like *Szene Hamburg*, *Hamburger Abendblatt*, and *Esotera*.

For more than twenty years, Barbara Simonsohn has been intensively involved with the topic of nutrition. She trained with the naturopathic physician Dr. Renate Collier to be a leader for seminars on acidosis and for fasting. She first became a whole-foods vegetarian and then changed her diet to vegan raw fruits and vegetables according to the principles of Natural Hygiene, represented by Marilyn and Harvey Diamond and David Wolfe, among others.

After working at the Hamburg University as a scientific assistant for several years, Barbara Simonsohn completed her training to be a teacher of the authentic Reiki® in 1984 with Dr. Barbara Ray in the USA, with Dr. Willy Fraefel in Switzerland and with Gary Samer in Australia. Since then, she holds lectures and seminars in the USA and Europe on learning this simple and effective technique for deep relaxation, stress reduction, strengthening the immune system, and personal development in all seven degrees.

Barbara Simonsohn's son Michael was born in 1988 and her daughter Freya was born in 1994. She lives with her children in a home with a large garden in Hamburg, Germany. Here she not only has flowers but also organically grown vegetables and fruit, including mountain papayas, kiwis, and—most recently—stevia plants.

In addition to seminars on the authentic Reiki®, movement, acidosis therapy, The Five Tibetan Rites, and nutrition, she has written about these topics in many German-language magazines such as *Koerper, Geist und Seele Hamburg, Bio, Natuerlich leben, Natur & Heilen, Esotera, Wegweiser, Lichtgarten, Der Spatz,* and *Natur.* She hosts "Tropical Fruit Feasts" with an accompanying lecture on a regular basis.

Together with the English healer Alexander Aandersan, Barbara Simonsohn organizes events on activating the powers of self-healing and harmonizing relationships. She also organizes seminars in Germany with Neale Donald Walsch, author of *Conversations with God.*

Barbara Simonsohn is also involved in the Hamburg organization *Hilfswerk Haiti* as a developmental-aid helper. She holds women's seminars in Haiti that include planting fruit trees and plans to soon start a stevia project for improving the financial situation of people who live in the countryside there. Information about current projects and events with Barbara Simonsohn, as well as her latest articles, can also be found on the Internet (www.barbara-simonsohn.de).

Index

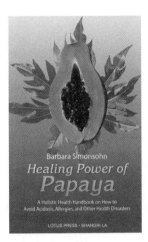

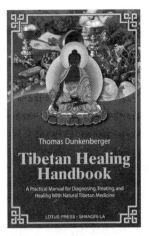

Barbara Simonsohn

Healing Power of Papaya

A Holistic Health Handbook on How to Avoid Acidosis, Allergies, and Other Health Disorders

Best-selling German author Barbara Simonsohn shares knowledge that native peoples from all over the world have successfully practiced for centuries. The "power fruit" papaya is virtually a universal remedy with a large spectrum of anti-inflammatory effects against many health disorders and diseases. Today, scientific research has confirmed all aspects of this empirical medicine.

And since the papaya is one of Mother Earth's best-tolerated, enjoyable foods, the author has provided numerous interesting food and cosmetic recipes. Valuable tips on a healthy diet and lifestyle complete the book.

Healing Power of Papaya also has an A-Z section, making it an excellent reference work for anyone who wants to use the papaya to become *healthy and fit*—and stay that way.

224 pages · $15.95
ISBN 0-914955-63-2

Thomas Dunkenberger

Tibetan Healing Handbook

A Practical Manual for Diagnosing, Treating, and Healing with Natural Tibetan Medicine

An introduction to one of the oldest healing systems: Tibetan natural medicine—comprehensive and easy to understand.

The author informs you about the essential correlations and approaches taken by the Tibetan science of healing. It describes the entire spectrum of application possibilities for those who want to study Tibetan medicine and use it for treatment purposes.

Tibetan Healing Handbook discusses the fundamental principles of health and causes of disease. These include non-visible forces and biorhythmic-planetary influences; classic Tibetan forms of diagnosis, the foremost of which are pulse and urine examination, advice on behavior and healing approaches to dietary habits, as well as the accessory therapeutic possibilities of oil massages, moxabustion, hydrotherapy, humoral excretion procedures, and famous Tibetan remedies.

240 pages · $15.95
ISBN 0-914955-66-7

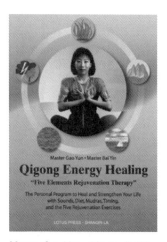

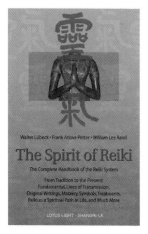

Master Gao Yun · Master Bai Yin

Qigong Energy Healing

Five Elements Rejuvenation Therapy

The Personal Program to Heal and Strengthen Your Life with Sounds, Diet, Mudras, Timing, and the Five Rejuvenation Exercises

Qigong energy healing means strengthening the life energy with sounds, the right timing and diet, with certain mudras, and with the five rejuvenation exercises. These five elements are the basis for revitalizing the energetic field of the body and mind. With the help of *Qigong Energy Healing*, everybody can find out his own "qi code", the best time of the day, the right sounds, the mudras, and the vitalizing five elements rejuvenation exercises that correspond to his personal type. These exercises are short, meditation movements that can be performed effortlessly. They cleanse the meridians, so that the qi can flow freely. Also suitable for those who have no previous experience with qigong.

80 pages · $14.95 · full color
ISBN 0-914955-69-1

W. Lübeck / F.A. Petter / W.L. Rand

The Spirit of Reiki

The Complete Handbook of the Reiki System

From Tradition to the Present: Fundamental, Lines of Transmission, Original Writings, Mastery, Symbols, Treatments, Reiki as a Spiritual Path in Life, and Much More

Never before, have three Reiki masters from different lineages and with extensive background come together to share their experience.
A wealth of information on Reiki never before bought together in one place. The broad spectrum of topics range from the search for a scientific explanation of Reiki energy to Reiki as a spiritual path. It also includes the understanding of Dr. Usui's original healing methods, how Reiki is currently practiced in Japan, an analysis of the Western evolution of Reiki, and a discussion about the direction Reiki is likely to take in the future.

312 pages · $19.95
150 photos and b/w illustrations
ISBN 0-914955-67-5

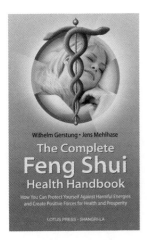

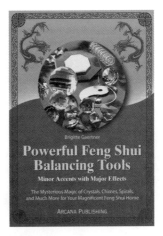

Wilhelm Gerstung and Jens Mehlhase

The Complete Feng Shui Health Handbook

How you can Protect Yourself Against Harmful Energies and Create Positive Forces for Health and Prosperity

The authors are experienced Feng Shui practitioners and consultants. They explain how the invisible energies of Feng Shui can be directly measured and evaluated using a tensor (single-handed dowser) or pendulum. This means that you can use Feng Shui to understand many health problems by relating them to energy imbalances.

This fascinating handbook provides a wealth of graphics and practical information, which help design every home in such a way that it becomes a source of energy, allowing everybody to relax and re-energize himself. The authors integrate their many years of research and extensive knowledge of energies in the home, and particularly the sleeping area, with the Western science of underground watercourses and grids.

248 pages · $16.95
ISBN 0-914955-60-8

Brigitte Gaertner

Powerful Feng Shui Balancing Tools

Minor Accents with Major Effects

The Mysterious Magic of Crystals, Chimes, Spirals, and Much More for Your Magnificent Feng Shui Home

Powerful Feng Shui Balancing Tools is a standard work, based on the traditional Chinese knowledge, a book that exclusively presents these mysterious accents with powerful effects. A balancing tool consciously placed in the right location of your home exerts concealed positive Chi powers which harmonize the area of its influence, improving the quality of your life, by giving you inner peace, comfort and a long-lasting health.

Powerful Feng Shui Balancing Tools provides a wealth of lovely colored illustrations and pictures, which help you choose the proper accents to energize and clear your home from clutter in such a way, that it becomes a source of flowing Chi.

96 pages · 108 photos · $14.95
ISBN 0-910261-20-2
ARCANA PUBLISHING

Herbs and other natural health products and information are often available at natural food stores or metaphysical bookstores. If you cannot find what you need locally, you can contact one of the following sources of supply.

Sources of Supply:

The following companies have an extensive selection of useful products and a long track-record of fulfillment. They have natural body care, aromatherapy, flower essences, crystals and tumbled stones, homeopathy, herbal products, vitamins and supplements, videos, books, audio tapes, candles, incense and bulk herbs, teas, massage tools and products and numerous alternative health items across a wide range of categories.

WHOLESALE:

Wholesale suppliers sell to stores and practitioners, not to individual consumers buying for their own personal use. Individual consumers should contact the RETAIL supplier listed below. Wholesale accounts should contact with business name, resale number or practitioner license in order to obtain a wholesale catalog and set up an account.

Lotus Light Enterprises, Inc.

P. O. Box 1008
Silver Lake, WI 53170 USA
262 889 8501 (phone)
262 889 8591 (fax)
800 548 3824 (toll free order line)

RETAIL:

Retail suppliers provide products by mail order direct to consumers for their personal use. Stores or practitioners should contact the wholesale supplier listed above.

Internatural

33719 116th Street
Twin Lakes, WI 53181 USA
800 643 4221 (toll free order line)
262 889 8581 office phone
WEB SITE: www.internatural.com

Web site includes an extensive annotated catalog of more than 10,000 products that can be ordered "on line" for your convenience 24 hours a day, 7 days a week.